Hydrotherapy:
Simple Treatments
For Common Ailments

By

Clarence Dail, M.D.
and
Charles Thomas Ph.D.

TEACH Services
Brushton, New York

INTRODUCTION

Rather than going to the medicine cabinet for a drug to take for such common ailments as the common cold, as for a headache, nervousness, sleeplessness and many other ailments would it not be better to use effective treatment that does not leave some foreign chemical in the body? This manual describes step by step such treatments using simple methods. Although these methods are simple, your physician should be informed of your actions.

First, let us consider the healthy human body. All the organs work in harmony with each other, they support each other. They all contribute to the total health. Each organ works more or works less according to the need. Thus:

1. As we breathe, the lungs obtain oxygen from the air around us and furnish it to the blood. When we work hard we breathe more rapidly and deeply, since the need is greater.

2. The heart pumps our blood containing the oxygen it got from the lungs through the arteries to all the organs including the muscles. Just like with the lungs when we work hard our heart pumps more rapidly and more deeply.

3. As the blood flows through the stomach and intestines, it picks up nutrition that has been prepared by digestion of food that we have eaten. Just like with oxygen, the nutrition in the blood is carried to all the organs.

4. Now, the oxygen is used and the nutrition is utilized ("burned") by the life processes (metabolism) of all the organs and every living cell. This action results in waste products ("smoke").

5. These waste products are carried in the blood by the blood vessels to the kidneys and from there into the urine. Furthermore, the "burning" (metabolism) process also produces carbon dioxide (as in "smoke") which is returned to the lungs and from there into the air surrounding us.

Our brain is one of the organs which is serviced by the blood. In fact, it is the most important organ we have. It is the control center for the whole body. It communicates with every part by sending "messages" through the spinal cord and through the many nerves. In turn, it receives information from every part of the body. It communicates with the outside world through the eyes, ears, nose, mouth and muscles. It is with the brain that we think. It is really in the brain that you and I are persons and have our individual personalities. Here we learn. Here we develop character.

How did this wonderfully designed human being ("mechanism") of ours come about? By evolution? No! It was created by God in His very image. It was so designed that it could reproduce itself over and over again from generation to generation through the many ages—through the times of the long-lived pre-flood ancestors of ours, through the patriarchal times, through the Roman period, throught the Dark Ages. Even now after so much sin and disease we can see the wonderful handiwork of God in our bodies.

As first stated, all the organs of the body work in harmony with each other, they support each other. If one organ is sick or injured, all other organs suffer, the whole body is sick. We cannot live without any of the following: the heart, the lungs, the liver, the pancreas, the kidneys, the stomach together with the intestines, and of course without the brain and the nerves. Furthermore, we cannot move, speak or do anything without the muscles.

The smallest and fundamental building block of all organs is the cell. The cell is so small it cannot be seen but with a microscope. Each has a special work to do. But all have certain things in common:

1. They all come from previously living cells.

2. They all use oxygen to burn food, for heat and energy for the processes of life.

3. They produce waste products such as carb-on dioxide like smoke from a fire.

4. They all need water to live.

5. They grow and repair themselves.

6. They reproduce--make more cells (with a few exceptions).

7. They all eventually die.

8. They all have characteristic structure, some extremely complex.

9. They are really chemical factories.

10. Every cell in my body has an imprint which is different from every cell in your body. This imprint is due to the genes we get from our father and mother. The ovum cell from my mother united with the sperm cell of my father to form my original cell. This original cell has all the information needed for the construction of my body; to form all my parts, to make me look like myself, to produce the color of my hair, to make me act like myself differently than you act. Oh, how marvelous is my Creator!

Each of the innumerable billions of cells in my body have all these characteristics. Now the cells are grouped together for specific functions and thus can be more efficient. Thus, a small group of cells can form a gland such as a sweat gland. A larger group can be organized into an organ, such as the heart. Furthermore organs can function together into a system such as the circulatory system. We may look at the cell as one person in a large crowd; we may think of a gland as a family of persons in that group, of an organ as a community of families, of a system as a city. Just as the city with its mayor, the community, the family, and the individual have support systems or utilities or services such as water lines, sewer systems, gargage disposals, roads, telephone, banks, stores, etc. so the body has to have support systems. These include the digestive system for food, the respiratory system for oxygen, the circulatory system for transportation throughout the body, the excretory system for getting rid of wastes and finally the nervous system for control. As previously pointed out, the nervous system, the head of which is the brain, is what makes you and me persons. More that any other system, the brain has to have support from all systems. The welfare of the brain, of our ability to think, to reason, to live a correct life depends on the proper functioning of all the systems. How important it is for me to take good care of these support systems of my body! Not only should I do all I can to have good healthful habits but my very attitude and frame of mind strongly influences the function of all the organs. "A merry heart doeth good like a medicine: but a broken spirit drieth the bones." Proverbs 17:22.

In spite of the many attacks of disease, of poisons, of injuries and in spite of changes in the temperature of our environment, our bodies are so constructed that they protect us in remarkable ways. Each organ, in fact, all cells of our body, are surrounded by a life-giving fluid which contains just the right kinds and amounts of chemicals and have the right temperature for the best function. For instance:

1. Suppose a common cold virus attacks us. We may get a sore throat and generally feel miserable. A fever develops. This is evidence that a war within our body is going on. With the increase of temperature all the chemical actions increase and become more effective.

At the same time, life processes also increase. Thus the ability for the white blood cells to attack and kill viruses and bacteria is increased. The body has reacted and the infection is overcome.

2. Suppose I hurt my foot. The foot may become inflamed and warmed. There is a reaction to improve healing, since the healing is helped with increase in temperature.

3. If I step outdoors into the cold, I may begin to feel chilly and start to shiver. That is a reaction. There is less blood going to the skin and thus the warmth in the body is saved. Also, more heat may be produced in the muscles by shivering, thus body temperature is preserved.

These three examples show how the body reacts to anything that might keep it from being normal.

Because of reaction:

1. The body temperature is kept close to 37 degrees Celsius (98.6 F.) even when in a cold room.

2. The oxygen and the carbon dioxide in the blood are kept at normal values even though I may be sleeping or exercising.

3. The blood sugar is maintained within a normal range even though I have just eaten a heavy meal.

4. The blood pressure is kept at a reasonable range even though I might have gotten quite angry.

5. A wound has healed so that after a month following the injury there is only a small scar.

There are many more such functions (scores more) of the body that are kept normal in the healthy body by reaction to many obnoxious influences about us. You may have had a laboratory blood test done. On looking at the report slip there might be seen as many as twenty things you could be tested for (such as hemoglobin, blood sugar, number of red blood cells, etc.). All of these listed on the report sheet are usually given a normal range. If the reported value is above or below the range shown, there is an abnormality, this might mean disease. The body reacts to maintain these normal ranges. Failure of reaction may mean disease or even eventually death.

The ability of the body to react may be improved by the use of water treatments as it is made to react to the heat and to cold applications. As we describe the use of the different treatments we shall refer to these reactions.

Now there is another effect of hot or cold water treatments that must be realized. This principle applies to all living creatures and even to all chemical reactions.

Note the following:

1. The "cold blooded" lizard moves very slowly when the weather is cold; it moves rapidly when the weather is hot.

2. We keep food from spoiling by placing it in a cold refrigerator.

3. Eggs are placed in a warm incubator so that the chicken will hatch.

4. We cook food so that it can be eaten and digested better.

5. A mountain skier when caught in an avalanche may die from being frozen.

6. Wood burns better when placed in a very hot stove than when starting a fire in a cold stove.

These examples illustrate the principle that all life is more active as the living being is warmer, as long as the increased heat does not cause damage. The activity is slower with cooling as long as the lower temperature does not injure. This principle is also made use of in giving simple water treatments. Thus there is the direct action of hot or cold water as it is applied to the body but as previously described, the reaction to this direct action in the normal body attempts to counteract that direct action. Thus if a cold wet cloth is applied to the skin, there is the immediate cooling of the skin and immediately the normal body reacts to fight against that cold by increasing the circulation to warm the skin.

As the different treatment methods are described in the following pages, we shall show the benefits which are to be obtained by the direct effect or by the reaction. Both effects are usually present, one of which is stronger. These effects help the body in its efforts to maintain and regain normal function and health.

Please now refer to the table of contents. The treatment methods are listed under two headings. The first are those treatments that are commonly combined for the best results. The second are those that are usually given separately. This second group is again divided into local and general treatments. The treatments are numbered for reference.

TABLE OF CONTENTS

III SIMPLE RATIONAL METHODS

TREATMENT ONE

HOT FOOT BATH

The hot foot bath is one of the local water baths (see treatment #11) which has a special use and is therefore described here. It is usually combined with treatments 2, 3, 5, 9, and 10 and may be used any time it is desired to warm the patient.

Purpose and Effects:
1. To provide local and reflex increase in blood flow through the feet and entire skin surface producing decongestion in internal organs and brain (derivative effect).
   a. to relieve congestive headache
   b. to relieve chest congestion
   c. to relieve pelvic congestion
2. To provide general warming of the body.
   a. to prepare patient for general applications of heat
   b. to prepare patient for tonic procedures
   c. to produce sweating (when prolonged)
   d. to help prevent or abort a cold
3. To aid relaxation and comfort.
4. To provide a treatment for local inflammation of the feet.
5. Increase white blood cell activity.

Indications:
1. Congestive headache
2. Chest congestion
3. Pelvic congestion
4. Preparation for other treatments

1

5. Warm the body
6. To stop nose bleed
7. Aid relaxation and comfort
8. Common cold

Cautions - Contraindications:
1. Circulatory disturbances
2. Impaired sensation
3. Any condition where circulation in feet and legs is poor (diabetes, vascular disease.)

Equipment:
1. Foot tub or container large enough and deep enough; five gallon can or dish pan may be used
2. Thermometer, if available; if not, test water with elbow; temperature 103°–110° F.
3. Sheet or bath blanket
4. Turkish towel, cold compress if needed
5. Material for protection of bed (rubber sheet or plastic)
6. Pitcher or dipper to add hot water

Treatment:
1. The patient can be lying or sitting.
2. Have the patient properly draped.
3. Have water temperature 103°–104° F. (39½°– 40° C.) and deep enough to cover ankles.
4. Assist the patient to place his feet in the tub. Place your hand under his foot and into the water first to make sure the water is not too hot.

5. Be sure the drape covers the tub.
6. Add hot water from time to time to increase the temperature gradually to 110° F (43½° C). of the hot foot bath. But make sure you remove the feet first before adding the hot water. Feel the temperature of the water before lowering the patient's feet in the water.
7. Continue 10 to 30 minutes. Check reaction for perspiration.
8. Use cold compress to head as needed.
9. When finished with treatment, pour cold or ice water over feet. Remove from tub, dry thoroughly, and cover well. Guard against any chilling.

       –OR–

   When finished with treatment, remove from tub, dry throughly, (omit cold or ice water), and cover well. Guard against chilling.
10. If patient is perspiring give an alcohol rub or other cooling treatment to whole body and dry thoroughly when finished.

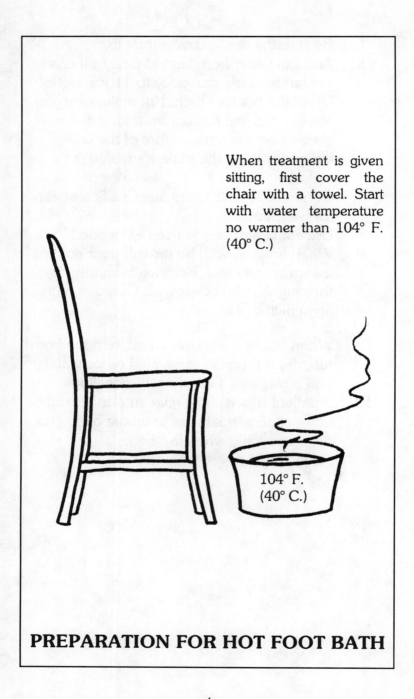

When treatment is given sitting, first cover the chair with a towel. Start with water temperature no warmer than 104° F. (40° C.)

104° F.
(40° C.)

PREPARATION FOR HOT FOOT BATH

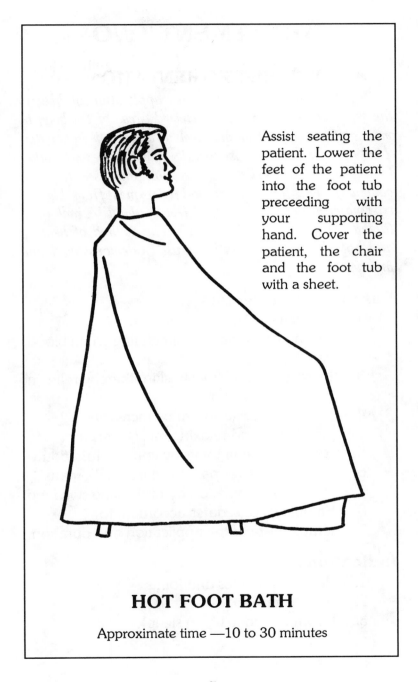

Assist seating the patient. Lower the feet of the patient into the foot tub preceeding with your supporting hand. Cover the patient, the chair and the foot tub with a sheet.

HOT FOOT BATH

Approximate time —10 to 30 minutes

TREATMENT TWO

THE HOT FOMENTATION

The hot fomentation is an application of heat to the skin over any of various selected areas of the body by means of a heated pad or towel wrung from hot water. The hot fomentation is usually combined with other treatments such as listed in section one (see table of contents). The fomentation pad is formed from blanket type material to be about 1 by 2 feet by about ½ inch thick (about 30 cm./60 cm./1 ½ cm.). The method of heating and applying the fomentation must be demonstrated and practiced.

Purpose and Effects:
1. To increase body temperature.
2. Promotes increase in circulating white blood cells.
3. Increases blood flow to skin, thereby relieving internal congestion.
4. Relieves muscle spasm by increasing circulation and relaxing muscle tension.
5. Relieves pain in joints by counter-irritation.
6. Reflexly relieves pain from internal organs.
7. Increases elimination by promoting sweating.
8. Stimulates or sedates according to temperature of the application and duration.

Indications:
1. Pain from nerves and joints.
2. Muscle tension.
3. Insomnia, (inability to sleep).

4. To warm the tissues in preparation for massage.
5. To prepare for a cold procedure.
6. Chest congestion from colds, bronchitis, pleurisy, (No cold used in treating pleurisy).
7. Nervousness - sedative to spine.
8. To produce sweating.

Contraindications:
1. Unconsciousness.
2. Paralyzed parts of the body.
3. Do not use on the legs or feet of a diabetic.
4. Edema and varicose veins and advanced vascular disease of the legs and feet.
5. Malignancy.
6. Tendency to bleed (hemorrhage).
7. Stomach and bowel ulcers.

Important Considerations:
1. Be sure the water in the hot foot bath does not burn the patient. Consider the age and vitality of the patient.
2. Always ask if fomentations are burning the patient. If they are too hot, dry the skin and put towel between skin and hot fomentation.
3. Be sure the patient is always properly draped.
4. Know the patient's condition before you start.
5. Always have the room warm before you begin treatment; make sure there are no drafts.

6. Remember that the duration and frequency depends upon the desired effect.
    a. Stimulant: applications should be short (3-5 minutes) very hot and followed by cold.
    b. Sedative: applications should be longer (6-10) minutes) with mild heat.
7. Be especially careful with thin or aged persons and children.
8. Avoid chilling.
9. Be careful not to spread an infection.
10. Keep towels under fomentations dry, moisture will increase the chance of burning the patient.
11. Parts where bone is close to skin surface are especially apt to burn, so keep extra towels handy to use to protect these areas more, if necessary.

Equipment:
1. Large wool blanket - 1
2. Sheet - 1
3. Pillow - 1
4. Large buckets - 2
5. Oral thermometer - 1
6. Towels - 10
7. Water thermometer - 1
8. Blood pressure cuff and stethoscope - 1 each (encouraged to have but not mandatory)
9. Fomentation pads and covers - 5 each
10. Large kettle (canning kettle works fine) - 1
11. Basin of ice water
12. Friction mitts

13.   One or two compress cloths

Preparation of the Fomentation:
1.   Boiling Water Method
    a.   Fold a large bath towel lengthwise and twist as much as possible; place middle three-fourths into the boiling water and let it become thoroughly soaked.
    b.   Lift out of water and pull ends hard away from each other to wring out all the water possible. Let it untwist by dropping one end and holding the other end.
    c.   Lay it over the dry towel placed on patient's body if the wet, hot towel is very hot.

-OR-

Place hot towels on the skin surface and quickly remove it to avoid burning; watch very carefully to lift the towel if heat is not tolerated. The towel will cool off rapidly. *Practice* this skill thoroughly *before* you work on your client.
    d.   Cover with another dry towel.
    e.   Repeat procedure 3 or 4 times. In between the hot towels, briskly wipe the body surface with ice-cold cloth and then blot the moisture quickly. It is the moisture that burns the skin, therefore the skin must be dry completely before the next application.
2.   Steaming Method

a. Soak completely and wring out 5 large bath towels or fomentation pads (made of cotton and wool) in water.
b. Place the towels or the pads on the grid of a large canner (32 qts.).
c. Place enough water in the canner below the grid and boil it for 20 minutes – towels or pads should not touch the water.

3. Micro-wave Method
a. Take large bath towel soaked in cold water; wring out all the water possible.
b. Place the single towel in a black plastic bag (garbage bag).
c. Place the bag in the micro-wave oven and turn on "high" for 4 minutes.
d. Quickly remove towel and use it on the body surface; if it is very hot, place a dry towel on skin area before using the very hot towel.

Treatment:

1. Take the patient's temperature and record it.
2. Take pulse and respiration and record them.
3. Take blood pressure and record it.
4. Have patient disrobe and put on patient gown.
5. Have blanket on bed or table then place sheet on top of blanket.
6. Have patient lie on sheet and wrap blanket completely around the patient exposing only the head.

7. Prepare the water in bucket for the foot bath, 104° F (40° C.). Fill the bucket only half full. Place your hands under the patient's feet as you lower them into the water. Completely wrap the bucket and the legs with the sheet and the blanket.

8. Apply one fomentation under the patient's back.

9. Apply two fomentations across the chest. Leave on for 3 - 5 minutes. When the fomentation becomes comfortable, that is the time to change.

10. Between changes give cold mitten friction and dry area.

11. Make 3-4 changes to secure a good reaction; the skin will become red in treated area.

12. Cool patient down with cool or cold wash cloth and cold mitten friction rub.

13. Dry patient thoroughly.

14. Cover patient and have him rest for at least 30 minutes.

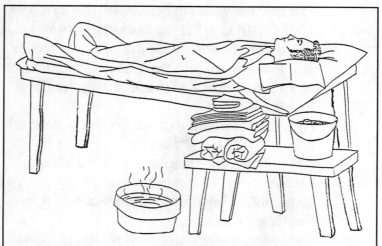

MATERIAL NECESSARY FOR
FOMENTATIONS TO CHEST AND BACK

Hot foot bath, 5 fomentations (1 for back, 2 for
chest, 2 in canner), 3 to 5 wool covers, 6 bath
towels, basin of ice water for cold compress.

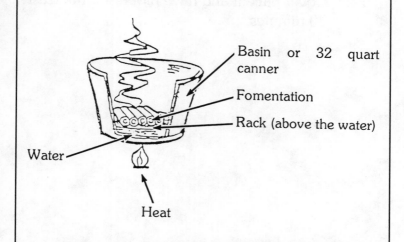

Basin or 32 quart
canner

Fomentation

Rack (above the water)

Water

Heat

HEATING OF FOMENTATIONS

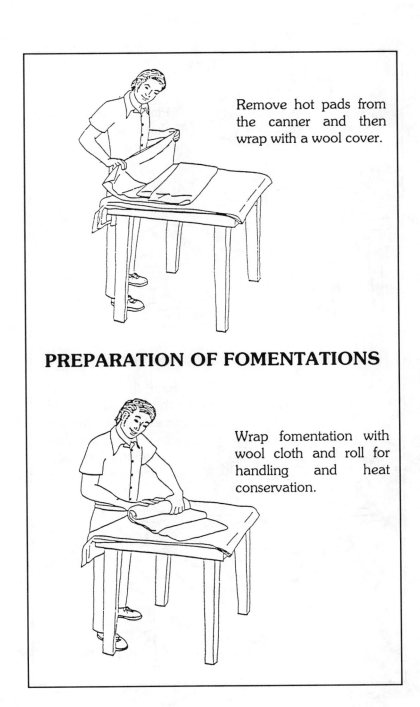

Remove hot pads from the canner and then wrap with a wool cover.

PREPARATION OF FOMENTATIONS

Wrap fomentation with wool cloth and roll for handling and heat conservation.

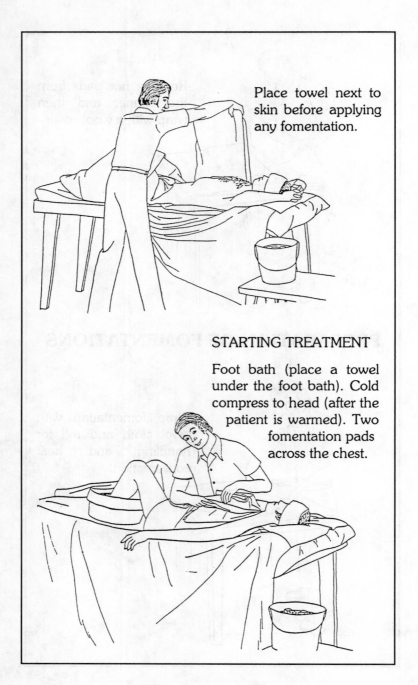

Place towel next to skin before applying any fomentation.

STARTING TREATMENT

Foot bath (place a towel under the foot bath). Cold compress to head (after the patient is warmed). Two fomentation pads across the chest.

When giving the hot foot bath in the lying position first cover the bed (or treatment table) with a waterproof sheet, then with a blanket and then a sheet.

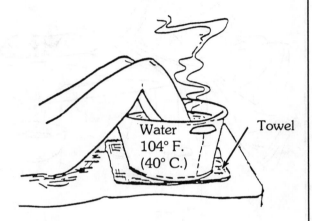

Water
104° F.
(40° C.)

Towel

Your hands into the water first before heel of patient.

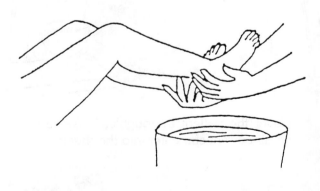

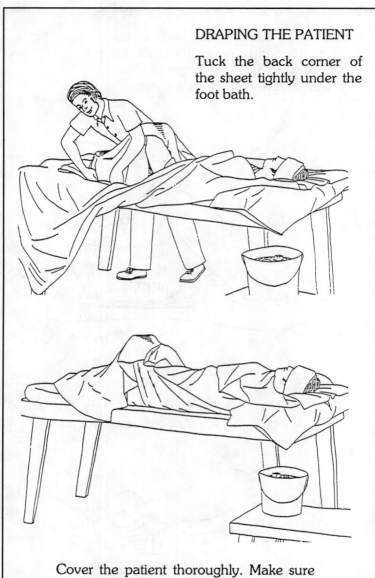

DRAPING THE PATIENT

Tuck the back corner of the sheet tightly under the foot bath.

Cover the patient thoroughly. Make sure no air current can enter into the sheets.

TREATMENT THREE

COLD MITTEN FRICTION

The cold mitten friction is an application of cold water together with friction to the arms, legs and body with the use of mittens. This treatment is given for its general stimulating effects after the body is well warmed up by some previous treatment such as a fomentation or a wet sheet pack (see treatment #9, p. 42). (see treatment #9, p. 42)

Purpose and Effects:
1. To stimulate circulation of the skin (dermis).
2. To increase the rate of blood flow.
3. To increase white cell activity and antibody production.
4. To stimulate neuromuscular tone.
5. To reduce fever.
6. Vasomotor tonic.

Indications:
1. Convalescence after fevers.
2. Hyperthyroidism (pre-operative & post-operative).
3. Nervous exhaustion.
4. To build up resistance to cold and general body resistance.
5. Sluggish circulation.
6. Generalized weakness and lack of endurance.

Contraindications:
1. When patient is chilled.

2. Skin lesions or eruptions on area to be treated.

Equipment
1. Two sheets or two bath blankets
2. Two mitts
3. Pail or large basin of cold water, temperature 40°–70° F.
4. Bath towels
5. Material for hot foot bath and cold compress for the head.

Procedure
1. Important Considerations
   a. Make sure the patient is warm, especially his feet.
   b. Do not expose more than one part of the body at one time, avoid chilling.
   c. Avoid skin lesions.
   d. The patient must be kept warm and dry after the treatment.
   e. Success of the cold mitten friction depends on the speed and vigor of the treatments.
   f. Best of all means for training to react to cold.

Preparation for Treatment
1. Protect the bed from dampness, use a bath blanket under the patient if necessary.
2. Explain the treatment and purpose.
3. Assemble the materials.

4. Water temperature 60°–70° F., lower temperature 1°–2° each treatment to 40°–50° F.

Treatment:
1. Make sure the patient is warm, especially the feet.
2. Do not expose more than one part at a time.
3. Avoid skin lesions.
4. Start with extremities first, then chest and finally the back.
5. Wring mittens quickly from cold water, and rub vigorously for 5-8 seconds.
6. Quickly cover part with dry towel and dry with friction.
7. Cover the area with dry bath blanket and proceed with the next body part.
8. Tonic or stimulating effects depend on:
   a. temperature of the water
   b. repeated dipping of mittens (1-4 times)
   c. the duration of the application
   d. the vigor of friction applied
9. Be sure the patient is warm and dry.
10. Have patient rest ½ hour.
11. The cold mitten friction may be part of another treatment such as the fomentation.

HOT MITTEN FRICTION

Same as "Cold Mitten Friction" only using hot water — hot as can be tolerated by person giving the friction.

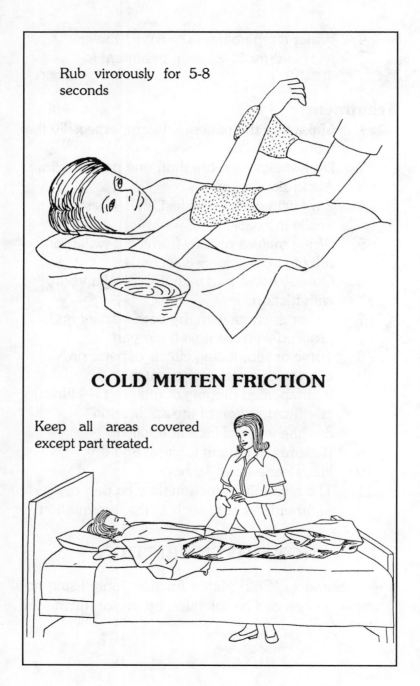

Rub virorously for 5-8
seconds

COLD MITTEN FRICTION

Keep all areas covered
except part treated.

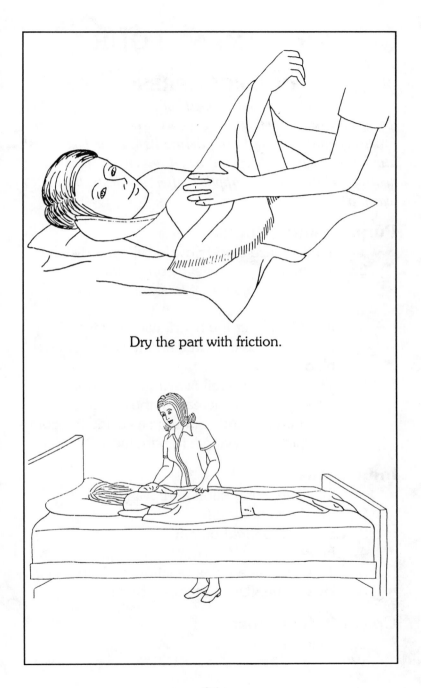

Dry the part with friction.

TREATMENT FOUR

COLD COMPRESS

The cold compress consists of a cloth wrung out of icy water and applied to various areas such as the forehead and over the heart. Before its use the body must always be warm, therefore when given as part of a heating treatment it is applied after the body begins to warm up.

Purpose and Effects:
1. To decrease blood flow locally and distally.
2. To prevent and relieve congestion.
3. For relief of pain due to swelling and/or injury.
4. If applied over the heart: will slow the heart rate, increase the force and raise the arterial blood pressure.
5. To increase the reflex action of thermal applications by increasing the difference between hot and cold such as using the cold compress following a fomentation.

Indications:
1. Swelling, congestion and/or injury.
2. Increased heart rate.
3. Shallow labored breathing.
4. Fever.
5. To stimulate a reflex reaction. (#5 above)
6. Headache. (Use with hot foot bath)

Contraindications:
1. Diabetes.

2. Skin disease.
3. Patients who cannot tolerate cold.
4. Patient who is chilled; wait until the entire body is warm.

Equipment

1. Compress may be a wash cloth or hand towel (terry cloth) cheesecloth, etc. (The size depends on the part to be treated.)
2. Basin for cold or ice water.
3. Plastic or rubber sheeting.

Procedure

1. Important considerations
    a. Some patients cannot tolerate moist cold over sinuses.
    b. Remember reflex effects of cold: concomitant vasoconstriction in opposite limb and reflex area.
    c. Keep bed dry.
    d. Do not drip cold water on patient.
    e. Do not let patient get chilled; especially watch when applying compress over a large area; use with hot foot or arm baths if possibility of chilling is present.
    f. Never cover a cold compress.
2. Preparation for treatment
    a. See that the patient is in a comfortable position.
    b. Have the room warm with no drafts.
    c. Protect pillow and bed with plastic.
    d. Assemble equipment.

Treatment:

1. Place compress in cold water and wring out just enough so it does not drip.
2. Apply and press firmly; if patient is sitting up while receiving treatment, compress must be long enough to be wrapped around head so it will stay in place, otherwise just across patient's forehead is adequate.
3. Renew frequently, every 1-5 minutes; have basin right beside you.

Completion of Treatment

1. Remove compress and dry skin thoroughly.
2. Make sure patient's hair is dry.
3. Pillows and bedding should be left dry (change if they are wet).

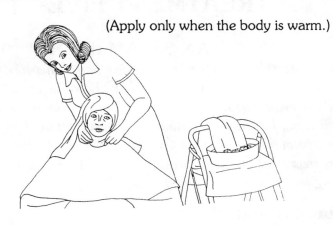

(Apply only when the body is warm.)

With many heating treatments, such as the fomentation already described, the hot tub bath and the wet sheet pack, described later, the cold compress is applied to the head after the body begins to warm up.

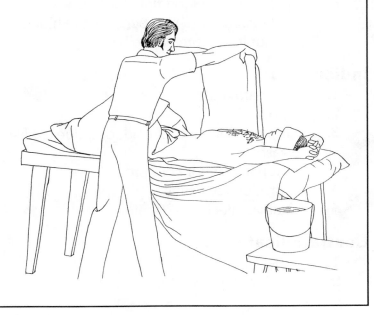

TREATMENT FIVE

RUSSIAN STEAM BATH

With the Russian steam bath the body is surrounded by hot very humid air. Because of this the body is heated by the surrounding heat all the more since heat is not lost by evaporation. Depending on the length of the treatment the body temperature will rise. As described, this treatment is given sitting; it may also be given in the lying position.

Purpose and Effects:

1. To increase body temperature.
2. To increase metabolism.
3. To induce sweating.
4. It will increase pulse rate.
5. It will increase blood pressure.
6. It will increase blood flow to skin.
7. It will increase the number of white blood cells out in the circulating blood.

Indications:

1. Rheumatoid arthritis.
2. Hypotension.
3. Symptoms of onset of cold, or influenza-like disease.
4. In preparation for cold procedures.
5. To produce sweating.
6. Sedative effect (15-20 min.)

Contraindications:

1. Diabetes.
2. Valvular heart disease.

3.   Emaciation.
4.   Advanced arteriosclerosis.
5.   High blood pressure.

Equipment:
1.   An old <u>wooden</u> chair
2.   Teakettle and hot plate
3.   Plastic cover (shower curtain sewed together does fine)
4.   3 towels (for draping around neck, over shoulders and over knees to keep plastic from touching directly on the skin).
5.   Hot foot bath and cold compress equipment.
6.   Ice bag.
7.   Wrist-watch with second hand.
8.   Drinking glass (water not cold); tap water.

Treatment:
1.   Heat the teakettle on a hot plate which has been placed under the chair with the spout facing to the back of the chair.
2.   Wrap the patient in a sheet. Have him sit on the chair.
3.   Give the patient a hot foot bath, about 104° F (40° C) to pre-warm him, apply a cold compress to the head.
4.   Remove the sheet, place a towel around the shoulders and neck.
5.   Drape a sheet or plastic cover around the patient's neck, covering the body from the neck down (like a tent) including the hot foot bath.

6. Check pulse frequently (if over 120/minute apply ice bag to the heart).
7. Encourage drinking of warm water to hasten sweating.
8. Duration: Tonic effect – 6 minutes; Sedative effect – 15 to 20 minutes
9. Conclude treatment by having the patient lie down, warmly wrapped, for a minimum of 30 minutes.

Cover the seat with a towel. Start the foot bath temperature at 104° F. (40° C.)

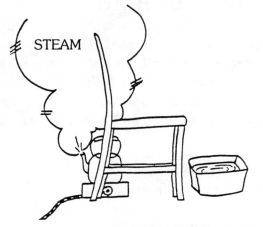

STEAM

(Take caution with the electrical cord).

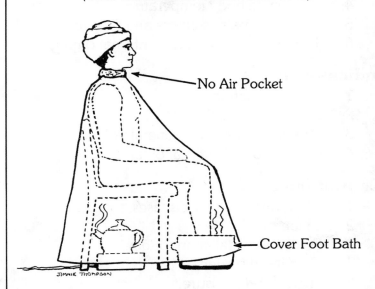

No Air Pocket

Cover Foot Bath

JIMMIE THOMPSON

Apply a cold compress to the head after the patient begins to warm up.

TREATMENT SIX

HOT TUB BATH

With the hot tub bath treatment the whole body is immersed in water except for the head. Here as with the Russian bath, except for the head, the body cannot control its temperature by sweating; but the body is heated more since there is direct contact with the water, and water has the property to carry much heat and conducts heat very well.

Purpose and Effects:
1. To increase blood flow to skin.
2. To increase metabolism.
3. To increase perspiration.
4. To elevate body temperature.
5. To relieve pain, stiffness and fatigue.
6. To relieve congestion of internal organs.

Indications:
1. Poor circulation.
2. Pain.
3. Muscle stiffness and general fatigue.
4. Congestion of internal organs.

Contraindications:
1. Heart and valvular diseases.
2. Diabetes.
3. Diseases of malignant origin.
4. Vascular disorders.
5. High blood pressure.

Important Considerations:
1. Aged or frail people will not tolerate hot bath well.
2. If patient is on medication consult physician first.
3. If dizziness or faintness develops, STOP at once.
4. Never leave the patient alone.

Equipment:
1. Bath thermometer
2. 2-3 bath bowels and bath mat
3. Basin of ice water
4. 2 wash cloths or compress
5. Shower cap to protect hair
6. Rubber ring or folded towel for patient to sit on
7. Folded bath towel for head pillow
8. If prolonged:
   a. Ice bag
   b. Cool fluids to drink

Treatment:
1. Fill tub 2/3 full of hot water – 104° F. (40° C.).
2. Assist patient into tub. Make comfortable with a pad or folded towels under hips and behind head.
3. Cover exposed body parts with a towel or cover tub with a sheet or light blanket.
4. Keep head cool with a cold compress.
5. The first treatment should elevate the body temperature only 1° F. (½° C.). The

duration of this treatment should only be 10 minutes.

6. Cool water to 96° F. (35½° C.), for about 5 minutes. Encourage exercise in the water.
7. With longer bath times and increased temperature always use an ice bag over the heart and give fluids to drink.
8. Check pulse regularly. Do not let pulse exceed 80 beats/minute.
9. Assist patient from tub. Remember, he may become dizzy or faint with exertion getting out of the tub.
10. Follow the bath with an alcohol rub or a cool sponge bath.
11. Dry thoroughly and keep patient warm.
12. Have patient rest for 1 hour after treatment.

Most homes in the U.S.A. have short tubs as illustrated here, so the patient cannot fully stretch out. This actually results in a safer situation because the upper half of the body is able to lose excess heat by conduction and evaporation of sweat. Thus there is less danger of over heating. There are, however, popular spas and mineral baths where people can be fully immersed. Overheating is a definite danger then.

Of course, as with any treatment causing general body heating, there should be applied a cold compress to the head as needed.

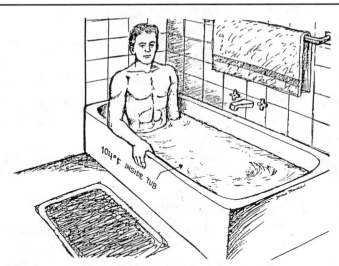

The heat application can be concentrated to the pelvic area by raising the knees out of the water. Water temperature may be raised as high as 109½° F. (43° C.). Such treatment may be helpful in pelvic conditions as bladder inflammation and dysmenorrhea. Do not use it during menstruation.

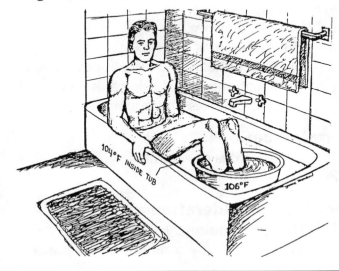

TREATMENT SEVEN

NEUTRAL TUB BATH

The neutral bath is neither hot nor cold. There is no increase in body temperature to produce increased body activity and there is no cold stimulus to cause reaction. Thus there is a quieting effect.

Purpose and Effects:
1. To relax the body.
2. To sedate the nervous system.
3. To provide sedation for patient with diseases of the heart and blood vessels who cannot tolerate hot and cold treatments.

Indications:
1. Cleansing.
2. Insomnia.
3. Nervous irritability, or exhaustion.
4. Anxiety.
5. Chronic diarrhea.
6. Multiple neuritis.
7. Diseases of heart and blood vessels where more extreme hot or cold cannot be used (such as diabetes and arteriosclerosis).

Contraindications:
1. Certain cases of eczema.
2. Great cardiac weakness.

Important Considerations:
1. The temperature: 94-97° F. (34½-36° C.) will vary with the condition of the patient,

season of the year, temperature of the room, etc.

2. If the patient is in the bath longer than 4 hours, lubricate the skin with a lanolin cream.

Equipment:

1. Bath thermometer
2. Turkish towels and bath mat if desired
3. 2 sheets and shower cp
4. Air pillow or folded towel for patient's head

Treatment:

1. Assist patient into tub, placing an air pillow or folded towel under head.
2. Cover exposed body parts with a towel or cover the tub with a sheet.
3. Instruct the patient to lie quietly and relax. Use a cold compress to forehead as needed.
4. Maintain constant water temperature.
5. Stay with the patient. Do not talk, except to keep patient quiet.
6. Duration: 15 minutes to 4 hours.
7. Assist patient out of the tub.
8. Dry quickly without friction or unnecessary rubbing. (Blot or pat gently).
9. Assist patient with dressing as needed.
10. Patient should have an undisturbed period of rest for at least 30 minutes.

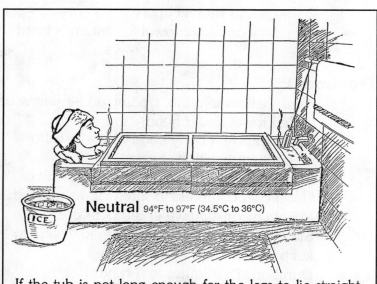

Neutral 94°F to 97°F (34.5°C to 36°C)

If the tub is not long enough for the legs to lie straight, the sedative effect can be had with the knees bent.

TREATMENT EIGHT

GENERAL COLD

COLD TUB BATH

The cold tub bath is a powerful stimulant. Use only in vigorous individuals.

Purpose and Effects:
1. With normal body temperature, stimulating and tonic.
2. With fever, may be cooling.
3. Increases white blood cell count in circulation.

Indications:
1. In the normal, gradual conditioning.
2. Common cold in an otherwise healthy person, following a strong heating treatment.
3. Fever.

Contraindications:
1. Debility as from a severe cold infection.
2. Cardiac disease.
3. Chilliness – heat first.
4. Menstruation.
5. Allergy to cold.
6. Severe diabetes.

Equipment:
1. Foot bath or other heating treatment.

2. Prepared bed with warm covering. Pre-warm bed with electric blanket or hot water bottles, etc.
3. Towels and friction mitts.

Treatment:
1. Make sure first that the patient is warm.
2. Explain the procedure.
3. May use a hot foot bath before (Treatment #1, p. 1)
4. Make sure that the bed is ready.
5. Fill the tub ⅔ with water the temperature being about 75° F. (24° C.).
6. Quickly assist the patient into the tub.
7. Rub vigorously with the mitts.
8. Duration: 10 seconds.
9. Having placed a towel on the floor for him to stand on, assist the patient out of the tub and dry quickly.
10. Quickly assist the patient into bed and cover warmly.
11. Remain well-covered for at least two hours or overnight.
12. May finish with a cold mitten friction (Treatment #3, p. 17)
13. The patient must dress warmly.

NOTE: When using the cold bath for the reduction of a high fever one must start with a temperature only a few degrees below the temperature of the body so that there is not a reaction to the cold. Such a reaction might even raise the temperature of the fever. The temperature of the bath is then slowly lowered. The temperature of the fever must be followed frequently. High fevers need to be treated under medical supervision, especially in the case of small children.

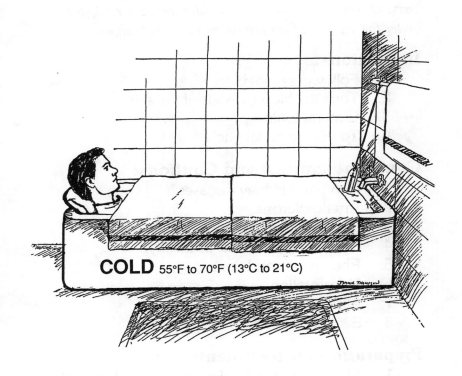

COLD 55°F to 70°F (13°C to 21°C)

COLD SHOWER

There is a shower in most American homes. It is in either a shower stall or over the bath tub. Like the cold bath, the cold shower is tonic. The temperature of the water from the cold pipes depends on the season and the climate. It may be as low as 50 F. (10 C.) or as high as 70 F. (21 C.). Thus the available stimulating effect may vary. Of course, by mixing hot water with the cold shower water the severity of the treatment may be changed.

Indications:
1. Following a hot bath.
2. Tone the blood vessels of the skin.
3. General tonic.
4. To overcome fatigue.

Contraindications and Cautions:
1. Heart and kidney diseases.
2. Arteriosclerosis.
3. Exophthalmic goiter.
4. Neuritis and nervous irritability.
5. Rheumatic conditions.
6. Menstruation.
7. Allergy to cold.
8. Severe diabetes.

Preparation for treatment:
1. Always be sure the patient is warm before the treatment.
2. There must be a non-skid surface on the floor of the shower.
3. Turn shower on and adjust the temperature.
4. Assist the patient into the shower.

Treatment:

1. At first, before the individual becomes accustomed to the cold, mix the cold with heat.
2. With each succeeding treatment lower the temperature about one degree.

Completion of treatment:

1. Dry well with friction.
2. Let the patient rest about 20 minutes before getting dressed. Avoid sweating in clothes.

Modification of the cold shower:

The tonic effects of the cold shower can be enhanced by alternating it with a hot shower. First adjust the hot phase to what is tolerated before the patient steps into the shower. Note the exact position of the hot faucet. Leave the heat on for one minute. Then turn off the heat for about 30 seconds. Turn the heat on to the exact position for one minute. Then the cold. Do this several times, ending with the cold.

TREATMENT NINE

WET SHEET PACK
(BLANKET PACK)

The wet sheet pack treatment consists of wrapping the patient with a sheet that has been soaked in cold water. Immediately after this the patient is further wrapped in a blanket. The reaction causes increased circulation and warming of the skin. Can be done using dry sheet.

Purpose and Effects:
1. To regulate the heating and cooling (evaporation) of the body so as to control the body temperature.
2. To cool a heated (fever) body.
3. To heat the body to sweating.
4. To quiet the nervous system.
5. To relieve internal congestion.

Indications:
1. Cooling stage: Antipyretic in fevers.
2. Neutral stage: Insomnia, mania, delirium, restlessness, nervous exhaustion, nervous indigestion, hypopepsia.
3. Heating and sweating stage: Alcoholism, nicotine poisoning, gout, bronchitis, common cold, influenza, jaundice, (measles, scarlet fever; to help develop the eruption).

Contraindications:
1. Diabetes or others with poor circulation.
2. Patients with severe colds or influenza.
3. Feeble persons.

42

    4.   Skin eruptions.

Equipment:
    1.   Material for a hot foot bath.
    2.   Material for a cold compress.
    3.   One or two woolen blankets.
    4.   2 large sheets.
    5.   Bucket of cold water (60-70° F.).
    6.   1 Turkish towel.
    7.   Fomentations, hot water bottle, or infrared
          lamp.

Treatment:
    1.   Pre-warm the patient with a hot foot bath,
          shower, fomentations or an infrared lamp.
    2.   Prepare the treatment table or bed.
          See: Page 46.
    3.   Soak sheet in cold water then wring sheet out
          as dry as possible. Spread out on table or
          bed. Patient must be undressed fully.
    4.   Have patient lie down on wet sheet with
          shoulders 3-4 inches below the top edge of
          the sheet.
    5.   Wrap the wet sheet around the body (under
          the arms) and tuck in on opposite side. Be
          sure the sheet is in contact with the skin.
    6.   Below the hips the sheet is wrapped around
          the leg on the same side.
    7.   Wrap the wet sheet from the other side over
          both arms and around the leg on that side.
    8.   Be sure no air pockets or loose places occur.
          Check the neck and arm areas.

9. Miter the blanket and wrap around the shoulders, arms and legs.

10. Wrap the other side in the same manner and tuck under the body.

11. Be sure the feet are thoroughly wrapped. If necessary place a hot water bottle to the feet, wrapped in a towel to hasten the warming reaction.

12. Cover the patient with additional blankets.

13. Place a turkish towel around the neck to protect the face and neck from the wool blanket and to exclude air.

14. Duration is according to the effects desired:
   a. Cooling stage: (used to reduce fevers)
      Leave a person in pack for about 20 minutes or until they feel a general glow and sensation of comfort and well-being.
   b. Neutral stage:
      Leave person in pack for about 1 hour or until person awakens.
   c. Heating stage:
      Leave person in pack until they start perspiring. Then it may be continued for 1 to 2 hours.

These treatment instructions together with the illustrations on the following two pages should be referred to in giving the wet sheet pack.

After completion of the wet sheet pack treatment (for stage 3 recommended, possibly for stage 1, but not for stage 2) it is desirable to give a cold mitten friction treatment (Treatment #3, p. 17).

If the patient does not react to cold even though he was previously comfortably warm, then the neutral stage (#2) and the heating and sweating stage (#3) can be accomplished giving the wet sheet pack as described only DO NOT wet the sheet. Leave sheet dry and follow all directions as above, or use blanket pack. Follow the instructions here given for the wet sheet pack but omit the wet sheet.

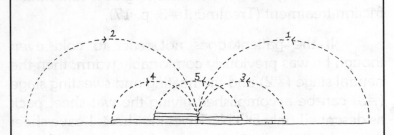

As instructed in treatment step #3 above, fold sheet lengthwise as shown and dip in cold water and wring "dry." Then lay the sheet on the blanket lengthwise and unfold it.

STEP-BY-STEP ILLUSTRATIONS DESCRIBING THE APPLICATION OF THE WET SHEET PACK

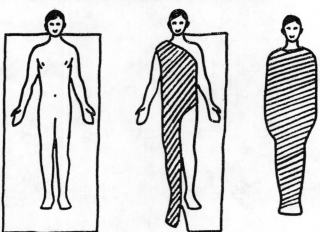

Then assist the patient to lie on the sheet face up.

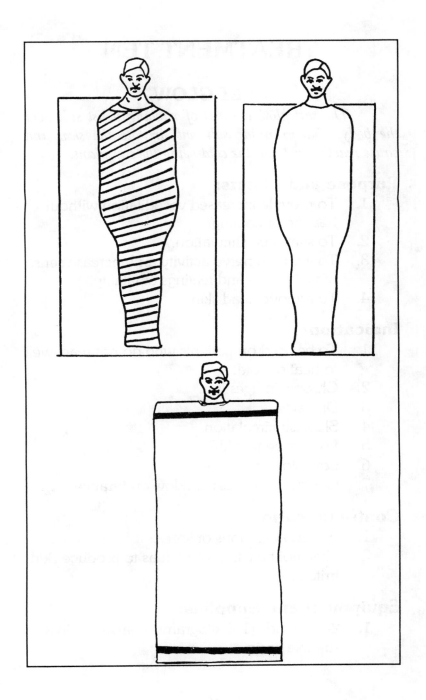

TREATMENT TEN

SALT GLOW

The salt glow consists of rubbing moist salt over the body. The granular salt will irritate the skin and cause reaction without the cold being the stimulant.

Purpose and Effects:
1. To provide increased vasodilation without heating or cooling.
2. To stimulate circulation.
3. To increase nerve activity and increase sense of well-being and feelings of vitality.
4. To remove dead skin.

Indications:
1. To be used on patients who do not react well to heat or cold.
2. Chronic indigestion.
3. Diabetes.
4. Sluggish circulation.
5. For frequent colds.
6. Low blood pressure.
7. General weakness and low endurance.

Contraindications:
1. Avoid skin lesions or sores.
2. Must not be used so often as to produce skin irritation.

Equipment and Supplies:
1. 2-4 pounds (1-2 kilograms) coarse salt in a suitable basin

2. Stool (only if patient needs to sit for the treatment)
3. Drape sheet and towels
4. Tub for foot bath
5. Available shower or pail for pail pour

Treatment:

1. Add just enough water to the salt to make it sticky (not too dry or too wet).
2. Prepare a hot foot bath at 104° F. (40° C.).
3. Have the patient stand in the foot bath.
4. Drape the patient with a sheet exposing only the part to be treated. Keep patient warm.
5. Pre-wet the part to be treated with water from foot bath.
6. Rub the part briskly with salt until the skin is pink.
7. Do all parts of the body in turn: arms and hands, shoulders, chest and abdomen, back, thighs, and legs and feet.
8. Remove the salt using a shower or pail pour.
9. Dry the patient well and keep him warm.

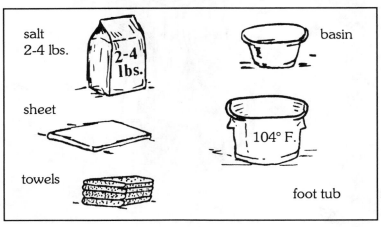

salt
2-4 lbs.

sheet

towels

basin

104° F.

foot tub

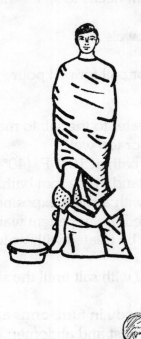

Keep the body warm and rub briskly.

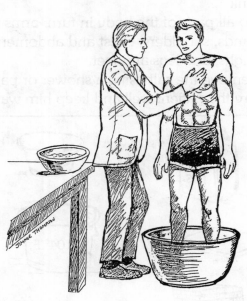

TREATMENT ELEVEN

LOCAL WATER BATHS

ALTERNATE HOT AND COLD LOCAL BATH

Purpose and Effects:
1. Alternate contraction and dilation of blood vessels.
2. Marked increase of blood flow locally and reflexly.
3. Increases metabolism and oxidation.
4. Hastens healing.
5. Increased white blood cell activity.

Indications:
1. Impaired venous circulation, indolent ulcers, (bed sores, varicose ulcer).
2. Infections, inflammation of the lymphatics.
3. Sprains, strains, trauma (after 24 hours).
4. Fractures.
5. Arthritis. (Rheumatoid and Osteoarthritis).
6. Congestive headaches, (treat feet).
7. Edema.

Contraindications:
1. Local malignancies (cancer).
2. Peripheral vascular diseases or diabetes.
3. Impaired feeling.
4. Tendency to hemorrhage.

Equipment:

1. Two containers large enough and proper shape to allow part to be treated sufficiently below surface of water.
2. Thermometer
3. Drape sheet or gown
4. Turkish towels
5. Cold compress for head
6. Disinfectant if needed
7. Pitcher to remove and add hot water
8. Means for heating water
9. Ice for the cold compress and the cold bath

Important Considerations Before Treating:

1. Usually a cold compress should be used for the head or even the neck. Use ice bag to the heart if the heart rate is over 80.
2. The hot water bath temperature should not exceed 110° F.
3. In the presence of possible peripheral vascular disease or diabetes, do not use water hotter than 105° F. Also avoid very cold in the cold bath.
4. Use a suitable disinfectant in the presence of any wound.
5. When adding hot water, cause it to touch your immersed skin before that of the patient.
6. If necessary, generally warm the patient before the treatment.

Preparation for the Treatment:

1. Assemble the necessary materials.
2. Have room warm and no drafts.
3. Position the patient and the containers so that the part treated can be easily immersed in either container.

Treatment:

1. Place part to be treated in hot water 104° F. (40° C.) for 3-4 minutes.
2. Place part in ice water or tap water — 45-70° F. (7-21° C.) for ½ to 1 minute.
3. While in cold water increase the temperature of the hot water to beginning temperature or slightly above. (Increase the temperature of the hot water each time the part is put in cold water but do not go above 110° F. (43° C.).
4. Check the pulse every 5 minutes, apply cold compress to neck and an ice bag to the heart if pulse exceeds 120 beats/minute.
5. Make 4 to 6 changes and end in cold. (In cases of rheumatoid arthritis, end in hot).
6. Dry thoroughly.

HOT LOCAL BATH

Aside from the effects described for the hot foot bath, the hot local bath may be used primarily for its local effects, and may be given to the arms and hands as well as to the legs and feet. The effects include increased circulation, increased tissue activity, increased healing, but tends to aggravate congestion if congestion is already present. (See Treatment #1, p. 1)

LOCAL COLD BATH

The local cold bath is given mainly for its local effects: Decreased tissue activity, decreased tissue inflammation, and also decreased tissue bleeding as in acute injuries.

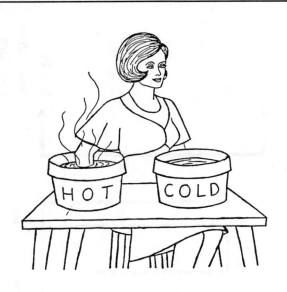

Suggested schedule on next page

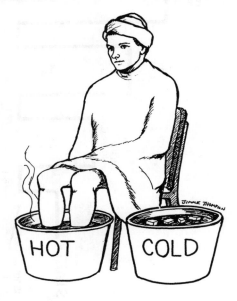

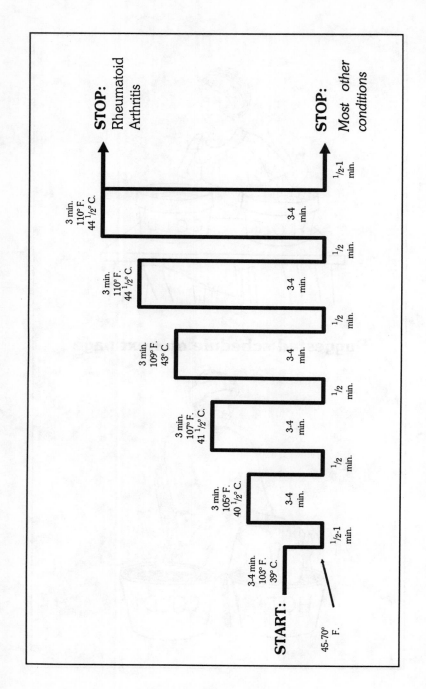

START:

45-70° F.

3-4 min.
103° F.
39° C.

½-1 min.

3 min.
105° F.
40 ½° C.

3-4 min.

½ min.

3 min.
107° F.
41 ½° C.

3-4 min.

½ min.

3 min.
109° F.
43° C.

3-4 min.

½ min.

3 min.
110° F.
44 ½° C.

3-4 min.

½ min.

3 min.
110° F.
44 ½° C.

STOP:
Rheumatoid
Arthritis

½-1 min.

STOP:
Most other
conditions

TREATMENT TWELVE

PARAFFIN BATH

Purpose and Effects:
1. Increases amount of blood flowing through the part and other effects of local heat.
2. The skin becomes soft, smooth and pliable, thus preparing the skin for massage.

Indications:
1. Arthritis
2. Stiff joints
3. Tendon repair
4. Sprains and strains
5. Inflammation of a tendon or tendon sheath
6. Old burns
7. Skin grafts
8. Following fractures

Contraindications:
1. Open sores on area to be treated.
2. Patients with diabetes (must use caution).
3. Weak elderly patients should be sure their hands do not touch the bottom of the container and are burned.

Properties of Paraffin:
1. Low specific heat.
2. Slow heat conduction.
3. Melting ability.
4. Easy to manage; reusable.
5. Inexpensive.

Equipment
1. Commercial paraffin bath or double boiler for home use.
2. Paraffin: 1 part mineral oil to 5 parts of solid paraffin (Parowax).
3. Dairy thermometer
4. Paint brush
5. Thin plastic and other material for covering

Treatment:
1. Wash part to cleanse from dirt and oils.
2. Show patient how to relax hands or feet so as to avoid cracking the paraffin "glove".
3. Have patient properly draped to keep him warm.
4. Make patient comfortable.
5. Temperature of the paraffin should be 128-130° F. (53-54° C.).
6. Dip body part 6-12 times (or paint with paint brush knees, elbows, back, etc.). Allow for paraffin to solidify (turns a dull white) before re-dipping.
7. After last dip wrap in plastic and cover with a towel to preserve the heat. Leave wrapped for 15-20 minutes.
8. If both hands are to be dipped, dip one hand first, complete treatment, wrap in plastic and then treat the other hand. The effect is prolonged by dipping both hands.
9. Remove the paraffin "glove" and use as an exercise "ball" for the fingers and hands; kneading and squeezing.

10. When finished, place the paraffin back in the tank. Give follow-up care as prescribed.
11. An alternate method of application is the use of painting the hot paraffin on the skin 6-10 times and then wrapping with the plastic and other cloth material.

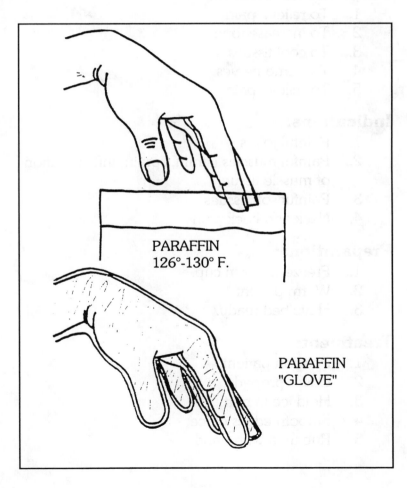

PARAFFIN
126°-130° F.

PARAFFIN
"GLOVE"

TREATMENT THIRTEEN

ICE MASSAGE

Ice massage consists of rubbing a block of ice over a skin area for the purpose of deep cooling of tissues. Penetration of the cooling effect is facilitated by the decreased circulation.

Purpose and Effects:
1. To relieve pain
2. To increase tone
3. To cool tissues
4. To numb nerves
5. To relieve pain

Indications:
1. Painful joints
2. Painful muscles (strain, sprain, inflammation of muscle tissue)
3. Painful soft tissues
4. Neck and back pain

Preparation:
1. Freeze water in cup.
2. Warm patient.
3. Have bed ready.

Treatment:
1. Position patient.
2. Cover properly.
3. Hold ice in mitt.
4. Smooth edges of ice.
5. Rub area with hand.

6. Rub Area with Ice.
7. Use circular motion.
8. Treat 5-15 minutes — 5 for thin tissue and 15 for deep tissue.
9. Patient Experience: The Four Stages —
    First – "Cold"
    Next – "Burning"
    Next – "Aching"
    Last – "Numbness"

Completion:

Have patient do a little mild, gentle motion – putting the part through all of its motion gently.

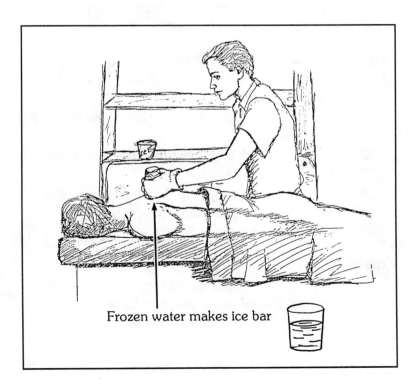

Frozen water makes ice bar

TREATMENT FOURTEEN

ICE PACK

Purpose and Effects:
1. To relieve pain.
2. To prevent swelling and black and blue tissue injury.
3. To decrease blood flow.
4. To decrease local metabolism.
5. To decrease deep tissue bleeding.
6. To decrease nerve response.

Indications:
1. Sprains, contusions, soft tissue injuries
2. Acute arthritis and bursitis

Important Considerations:
1. Observe the reaction of the skin to avoid skin damage.
2. Do not let the ice pack stay on more than 30 minutes.
3. Be sure that the ice pack is larger than the area to be treated.
4. Be sure that the patient is warm before the treatment is started, and is kept warm throughout treatment.

Equipment:
1. White heavy wool flannel (preferable stitched around the edge); a piece at least 12 x 12 inches for the shoulder or knee and 8 x 9 inches for the elbow or ankle.

2. 1 or 2 Turkish towels
3. Safety pins.
4. Plastic — 1 or 2 pieces.
5. Finely crushed ice or snow.

Procedure:
1. Important considerations:
    a. Observe reaction of the skin to avoid tissue injury.
    b. Apply pack for specified time, no more than 30 minutes at intervals of 2-4 hours as prescribed.
    c. Make sure rest of the body stays comfortably warm.
    d. Do not let wetness penetrate to the skin.

Treatment:
1. Prepare the ice pack by spreading a Turkish towel or flannel over a flat surface. Then spread finely crushed ice to make a layer about one inch (2 ½ cm) thick. Fold forming an envelope and pin the edges to prevent the ice from spilling out. Place an added layer of towelling or flannel between the skin and the pack.
2. Mold the pack evenly over the part being treated.
3. Do not let any water seep through the pack onto the skin.
4. Cover the pack with plastic and additional towelling.
5. May continue the treatment for 30 minutes and that at 2-4 hour intervals.

6. Make sure that the bed is dry at the end of the treatment.

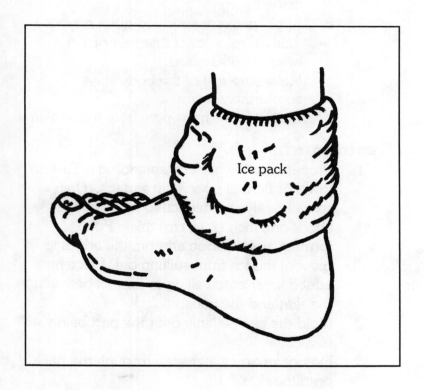

Ice pack

TREATMENT FIFTEEN

HEATING COMPRESS

The heating compress is an application of cold to a local area (throat, chest, abdomen joint, etc.) which causes a warming reaction. This warming effect is maintained by an immediate insulating covering applied over the cold application. This heating compress is left on for hours or over night.

Purpose and Effects:
1. First Stage – Cold
   a. Blood vessels narrowed
   b. Increased heart rate
   c. Increased respiratory rate
   d. Decreased metabolism
2. Second Stage – Heat
   a. Vasodilation
   b. Raised pulse rate
   c. Slight drop in blood pressure
   d. Increased sweating
   e. Oxygen consumption increased
   f. Fluid transfer across capillaries increased

Indications:
1. Heating chest pack
   a. Bronchitis (acute and chronic)
   b. Pneumonia, chest colds
   c. Early stages of influenza
   d. Cough
   e. Chest tightness after a cold
   f. Asthma
2. Heating throat compress

    a.   Pharygitis, chest colds
    b.   Laryngitis
    c.   Tonsillitis
3. Joint heating compress
    a.   To relieve joint pain and inflammation in rheumatic fever, chronic arthritis or synovitis (inflammation of a synovial membrane of a joint.)
4. Abdominal Heating Compress
    a.   Slow digestion
    b.   Constipation
    c.   Chronic appendicitis
    d.   Insomnia
    e.   Colic

Contraindications or Cautions:

1. Do not use moist compress when the patient is not able to warm it up. In its place you may use the "dry compress."

Equipment:

1. 1-2 thicknesses of loosely woven cotton cloth wide enough to cover the area and long enough for one circumference of the part (an old sheet is good).
2. Outer covering of the body part, wool flannel long enough to completely cover cotton cloth and extend ½ inch on each side.
3. Safety pins to secure compress in place.
4. Basin of water at temperature desired (usually tap water).
5. Towel to dry area with.

6. Wool (or Orlon) long-sleeved sweater —
   may need a long-sleeved cotton undershirt
   under the wool sweater to prevent skin
   irritation from the wool.

Procedure:
1. Important considerations:
   a. Wring cotton cloth so that it does not
      drip when applied.
   b. Apply compress smoothly and quickly
      to avoid chilling.
   c. Wrap snugly to exclude air and pin
      securely.
   d. Take care that compress is not so tight as
      to interfere with circulation, respiration
      or joint movement.
   e. Do not cover with plastic, this interferes
      with the reaction.
   f. Patient's ability to react to cold
      application is an important factor.
2. Preparation for treatment:
   a. Tell patient the application is cold but
      warms up by body reaction after the
      dry cover is in place.
   b. See that the patient is thoroughly warm
      before the compress is applied, give a
      hot foot bath if necessary.

Treatment:
1. Do not use the cold part of the heating
   compress when the patient does not react
   well to cold, and of course if he is yet chilly.

If he is chilly use an adequate method of heating first.

2. Immerse cotton cloth in cold water.
3. Wring the cloth out so it will not drip.
4. Apply the cold cloth and wrap snugly with flannel so air does not circulate.
5. Pin securely; do not spare the pins.
6. Cover chest and arms with a snug wool, long-sleeved sweater.
7. Leave in place for several hours or overnight.

Completion of treatment:

1. Remove compress, rub area quickly with a cold washcloth or alcohol.
2. Dry thoroughly; see that patient is warm and comfortable.
   NOTE: May be used as above only DO NOT wet the cotton (leave it DRY) and follow directions as above.

Heating Compress
for the throat or elbow

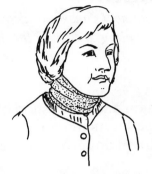 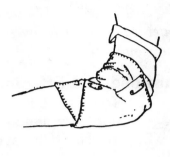

Heating Compress
for the chest

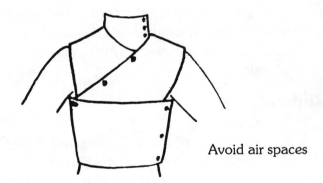

Avoid air spaces

I.   Wrap chest with cold sheet (or dry cotton-cheese cloth is good)
II. Cover cold sheet with wool flannel
III. Wrap neck with cold compress
IV. Cover neck compress with wool flannel
V.   Cover entire chest and arms with a snug turtleneck, long-sleeve, wool or orlon sweater.

TREATMENT SIXTEEN

STEAM INHALATION

The steam inhalation treatment consists of directed water vapor from a source of boiling water to the nose and mouth area.

Purpose and Effects:
1. To relieve inflammation and congestion of upper respiratory mucous membrane.
2. To relieve throat of irritation by moistening the air.
3. To relieve spasmodic breathing. (Asthma, Croup)
4. To loosen secretions and stimulate discharge of mucous from the throat and lungs.
5. To relax muscles and relieve coughing.
6. To keep mucous membranes from excessive drying.

Indications:
1. Coughing.
2. Congestion in lungs, nose and throat.
3. Throat irritation and dry throat.
4. Spasmodic breathing as in asthma and croup.
5. Loosen dry or thick secretions.

Contraindications:
1. Extremely young children or the very aged who may not be able to respond to heat.

Equipment:

1. Tea kettle with boiling water
2. Newspaper cone
3. Hot plate
4. Medication, pine oil, eucalyptus (optional)
5. Sheet
6. Umbrella

Procedure

1. Important Considerations
   a. Check inhalation frequently.
   b. Be careful not to burn patient.
   c. Be extra careful when treating children.
   d. See illustration on page 73
2. Preparation for Treatment
   a. Assemble equipment.
   b. Make sure there are no drafts in the room and that it is warm.
3. Treatment
   a. Fill tea kettle with boiling water; add medication to water.
   b. Carry to bedside and place on hot plate.
   c. Cover spout with a cone made of rolled newspaper in order to carry steam directly to person's nose and mouth.
      –OR–
      Place a towel over the head and catch the steam with the towel. If the patient is in bed, use an umbrella to make a tent (see illustration), place umbrella at head of bed, just above the patient's head and drape a sheet over it, making

sure the paper cone is under the "tent."
Do NOT completely enclose the patient.

    d.   Have patient breath slowly and deeply.

    e.   Continue for 30 minutes to 1 hour at least 2-3 times per day.

    f.   For continuous inhalation, place teakettle and hot plate on the floor without the paper cone. This will saturate the air of the entire room. Or use a vaporizer beside the bed.

4.   Completion of treatment

    a.   Make sure patient is warm and dry.

    b.   Encourage patient to rest for at least ½ hour after treatment.

This treatment may be given following other treatments such as fomentation to the chest.

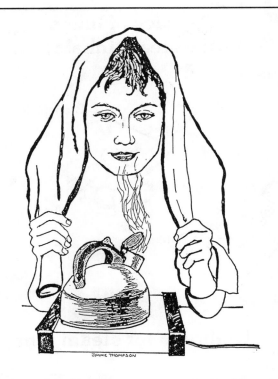

Paper funnel for steam inhalation

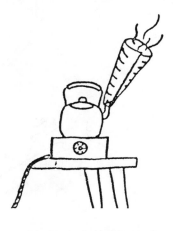

Air sacs of lungs during steam inhalation

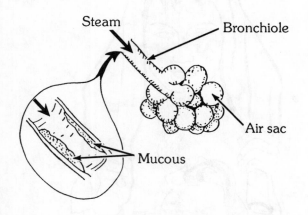

Steam

Bronchiole

Air sac

Mucous

Umbrella for steam tent

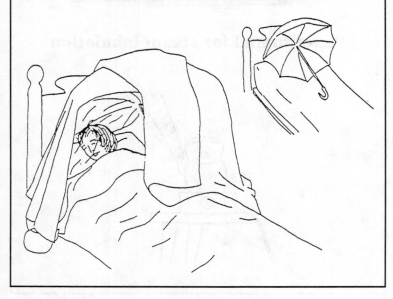

TREATMENT SEVENTEEN

CHARCOAL POULTICE AND SUSPENSION

Because of its physical structure charcoal has a very large surface area. A cube 2/5 inch (1 cm.) on each side has an area of a field about 33 yards (33 meters) on each side! Thus that amount has the ability to collect large quantities of liquids, gases, and dissolved chemicals. This quality is called ADSORPTION.

Indications:
1. To reduce inflammation
2. Local infections
3. Chemical poisons — internal and external.
4. Insect bites & stings
5. Diarrhea & gas — internal and external.
6. Wounds

Use as a Poultice:
1. Mix equal parts of flax seed meal and charcoal powder.
2. Add enough hot water to mix into a thick paste, like pudding.
3. Apply to clean muslin (thin cotton cloth) quickly to prevent cooling. The paste must be quite warm when applied.
4. Place on area to be treated. Cover with plastic and then wool cloth.
5. Pin in place (or use tape). Leave for several hours or overnight.
6. Remove; rub ice or very cold wet cloth over the area. Be careful if open wound.

7. Repeat if needed. Be sure to use a clean, new poultice – do not re-use.

Use in Suspension in Water:

1. Mix one tablespoon of the charcoal powder in a glass of water. May use the equivalent amount of tablets. The water should be hot.
2. After stirring, drink. May use two times a day.

Caution:

Charcoal should not be used over a long period of time as it will adsorb nutrition elements in the food as well as poisons and toxins.

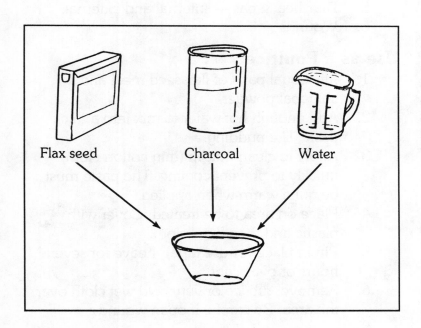

Flax seed   Charcoal   Water

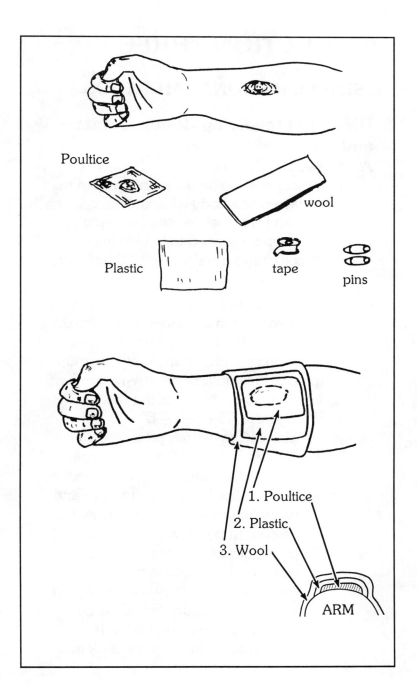

Poultice

wool

Plastic

tape

pins

1. Poultice
2. Plastic
3. Wool

ARM

SECTION THREE

SIMPLE RATIONAL METHODS

I. Disorders Involving Bones, Joints and Muscles

A. Bruises and Sprains

    1. Description—a bruise is an injury to the surface of the body without breaking the skin and is associated with swelling in the deeper tissues due to bleeding. A discoloration usually results: "black and blue."

    A sprain is an injury to a joint and its ligament due to an unnaturally forced movement beyond the normal range, resulting in severe pain, swelling, and internal bleeding. Bones are not broken and there is no break of the skin.

    2. What to do: "R—I—C—E"

      a. Elevate the injured part.

      b. For the first day after injury apply cold to the area, being sure to extend the cold application well above and below injury site. The cold used can be cold (not just cool) water (see p. 54) or towels wrung out in cold water and changed every 10 minutes. Keep injury cold until pain leaves. Take injury out of the cold and allow it to warm up by itself. When pain returns, put it back into

78

the cold. Remove when pain leaves. Continue this as often as necessary the first day.

c. After the first day, apply contrast baths (see p. 51) to the area or fomentation with ice rub 6 - 8 changes, 3 times a day.

d. Rest injured part—keep immobilized with supportive strapping.

e. On third day again apply contrast baths 3 times a day. Continue supportive strapping. (Should be applied by a trained person.)

f. On fourth day again apply contrast baths 3 times a day. The injured part may now be given very mild, gentle exercise if tolerated without pain. Continue supportive strapping.

g. Continue to apply contrast baths 2 times a day and supportive strapping until all tenderness is gone.

h. Gradually increase the gentle exercise until joint is normal.

i. The acronym R—I—C—E helps you to remember: Rest, Ice, Compression (strapping), and finally Elevation.

B. Whiplash Injury

1. Description—a sprain to the neck and results from an occupant of a car having his or her head snapped backward and rebounding forward when the car is hit from behind. Neck pain may be felt immediately at the time of impact or

after some time. Muscle spasm, local tenderness, and guarded motion, as well as swelling and headache, may result.

2. What to do:

a. Because of many complications, always see a physician and have him approve any treatment given; X-ray may be necessary.

b. First 24 hours:

(1) Apply cold (ice pack [see p. 54 & 62], cold compress, etc.).

(2) For 30 minutes on, 1 hour off, 30 minutes on, 1 hour off—alternating for 24 hours except while sleeping.

(3) Apply cold to neck area, front and back, well up into hairy area in back of head, upper back, tops of shoulders and upper chest.

(4) Use a hot foot bath with this so that patient does not get chilled (see p. 1).

c. Get a neck collar and use it right away, putting it on for that 1 hour between the ice pack treatments—also wear it all night.

d. Second day:

(1) Alternate hot and cold— fomentation [see p. 6] for 2-3 minutes, ice rub for 15 seconds, alternating at least 6 times) to the same areas 3 times a day.

(2) Wear collar all the rest of the time.

e. Continue second day procedure until healed. Then start gentle movements of the neck.

f. WARNING: Do not apply traction; it usually makes whiplash worse.

C. Muscle Strain

1. Description—Muscle strain occurs when a person makes an unusually forceful muscle contraction, as in an unexpected movement or improper use of muscle (as a sudden change of direction). There may be actual tearing of muscle or tendinous fibers. The most common sites are the back and calf muscles and usually associated spasm.

2. What to do:

At first, rest. With back strain, that means going to bed in the most comfortable position. Mild fomentation may help relax the spasm. After several days alternate hot and cold would help healing (p. 80; 2, d, # 1). Appropriate adhesive strapping can permit motion but must be applied by a trained person.

D. Bursitis

1. Description—A bursa is a sack that is lined with mucous membrane which secretes fluid, thus making the sack a lubricated pad. The bursa separates structures that move over each other, thus minimizing friction. If the bursa becomes inflamed there is pain on

movement. The pain may be due to swelling of the sack and pressure of the fluid. The shoulder bursa is the most common site of problems.

2. What to do:
   a. Mild heat may give relief, but, if there is appreciable distension, heat may aggravate the pain, since heat tends to cause further swelling.
   b. Ice pack (see p. 62) or ice massage (p. 60) tends to relieve the pain.
   c. After the part has become numb from the cold application, the part can be moved more freely. This should be done slowly and the range of motion carefully increased from day to day, always watching that the treatment does not cause more pain. In the more chronic condition, alternate hot and cold compresses (see p. 6) may encourage healing.

E. Fibrositis (Muscular Rheumatism)
   1. Description—an inflammation of the fibrous tissues in muscles, tendons and joint; the condition is common. The inflamed area may be felt as hardened nodules, bands or cords which are tender. The areas are painful and movement of that part causes increased pain. Common sites are in the neck, over the shoulder blades, and in the back. Associated headache is common. Inactivity, nervousness and poor posture

are causative factors, possible allergy and distant infections also.

2. What to do:
    a. Local heat as fomentations (see p. 6) or hot compresses (see p. 9).
    b. Massage over the part. Part of the massage may be what is called fibrotic or friction massage. This is heavy massage, the "nodules" being compressed with the operator's thumbs. This is painful, but gives relief. The operator needs to be trained to do this, but a family member can be taught.
    c. A good lifestyle is important.

F. Rheumatoid Arthritis
    1. Description—a chronic general disease affecting joints of the body which become inflamed. They swell, are painful, become stiff, and the structure of joints actually becomes destroyed. Deformity and crippling develop. There are acute and chronic stages. Although the specific cause is not established, contributing factors may include emotional stress, fatigue, injury, infection, exposure to damp, cold climate, and heredity. The patient needs to be under continuing care of a physician, so the following measures are only adjunctive.

2. Management
    a. Eat a wholesome, balanced diet—try to maintain normal weight; avoid food fads; eliminate all added sweets, fats and highly refined foods. Most arthritics seem to be sensitive to citrus fruit and juices; so if you are, avoid these.
    b. Adequate rest—early to bed and daily treatment naps.
    c. Moderate exercise—increase slowly if joints are not worse the following day, and if excessive fatigue is not produced.
    d. Daily sun baths—exposing as much skin as possible. Start with 5 minutes and gradually increase to ½ hour. Best time to sunbathe is before 10 a.m. and or after 4 p.m. in summer; and anytime in winter, but don't get a chill.
        (1) Contrast bath (p. 51)
        (2) Hot fomentations (p. 6)
        (3) Heating compress (p. 65)
        (4) Russian bath (p. 26)
        (5) Hot tub bath (p. 30)
        (6) Ice massage (p. 60)
        (7) Ice pack for acutely swollen joints (p. 62)
        (8) Paraffin bath (p. 57)
    f. For especially troublesome joints at night: rub with oil of wintergreen diluted one part to four parts olive

oil, cover with flannel, treat with
infrared lamp.

g. All joints should be put through
gentle but complete range of motion
several times daily.

h. Deep breathing exercises.

i. Measures to increase faith, and
combat tension and depression are
very important.

j. If contractures and severe joint
deformities have developed, the
doctor or physical therapist may be
able to devise specific exercises,
maneuvers, etc., to regain some
function.

3. Precautions—Mainly concerning
diagnosis as noted above, since many
diseases can cause painful joints. Close
cooperation with the doctor is most
important. Do not be overly vigorous
with exercises or treatments, since any
abrupt movement causes pain. One
must often be politely firm, however, in
encouraging the patient who is reluctant
to do anything. Generalized acute
flare-ups of the disease may require
hospitalization.

G. Osteoarthritis

1. Definition—a chronic condition affecting
especially the weight-bearing joints (such
as knees, hips, spine). There is a
thinning of the cartilage of the joints
(disks between and on surface of

adjacent bones) and even their destruction. There usually develops an overgrowth of bone or cartilage (lipping) along the edges of the joints. This is a condition of mechanical wear.

This condition is entirely different from rheumatoid arthritis in that it is very often associated with obesity and is due to "wear and tear" on the weight-bearing joints. It is seldom crippling, but may be quite painful. It is often complicated, especially in women, by osteoporosis, or the "thinning of the bones," due to calcium loss from too little exercise and from hormonal changes.

2. Management
   a. Weight reduction if obese—no treatment can succeed without this.
   b. Excessive use or exercise of involved joints should be avoided, but judicious exercise, slowly increased, is very helpful and is essential.
   c. Precautions: Severe and increasing pain on exercise may indicate extensive destruction of a joint, requiring virtual bedrest, specialized treatment by a physical therapist, aids in walking, or even surgery (possible artificial joints).
   d. Local treatment of individual joints essentially as described under Rheumatoid Arthritis. These

treatments can usually be more vigorous in osteoarthritis, and these patients will tolerate more heat and cold.

    e. Sun baths as under Rheumatoid Arthritis.

H. Joint Movement Limitation and Deformity

Taking care of the chronically ill, debilitated patient presents certain problems which are not so obvious. One of these problems is associated with the development of stiffness of joints and of soft tissues about the joints, as well as of deformities. Because of weakness there is little active movement and the tissues tighten. An example is development of bent and stiff knee and hip joints. The patient may find it more comfortable to lie with a pillow under the knees. Furthermore, it may be painful to move so stiffness also develops.

This problem can be prevented by proper positioning in bed and by movement of the joints throughout their full range done every day.

Although such a patient may never be rehabilitated, his care is much easier. Furthermore, deformed hips and knees increase the danger from development of pressure sores.

I. Backache
 1. Causes—Complaint of back pain is very
    common. The causes are numerous.
    The cause in a specific case may be
    obvious. The patient may have back
    pain following a fall or it may be
    associated with lifting a heavy object.
    Backache may occur in relation to time
    of menstruation or pregnancy. There are
    less obvious causes or contributing
    factors, such as arthritis, fibrositis,
    abnormal posture (e.g., poor sitting
    posture while driving), pelvic disease,
    disease of the kidneys, or a general
    disease such as influenza. Tension and
    emotional problems are important
    contributing cause of back pain. Finally,
    unless the cause has been determined,
    the possibility of cancer should be
    considered.
 2. Avoid Straining the Back—Before
    discussing treatment, we shall discuss
    how to avoid back strain associated with
    activities of daily living. These
    suggestions must also be considered in
    the care of a person with chronic back
    pain.
    a. When bending to pick up something,
       particularly when it is a heavy object,
       do not bend the back forward with
       the knees straight, but rather bend
       the hips and knees. Hold the object

close to the body; lift in front, do not twist.

d. If heavy work is necessary to move an object, call for help. In lifting, think out the best method. Use common sense.

c. In all your movements be sure of your footing and the stability of what you are about to step on. Stepping off a curb without planning for it can strain the back severely.

d. The height of a working surface (top of bench, table, kitchen sink) should be such that the back does not have to bend. Work with the hands close to the body.

e. Stand, walk and sit with head high, chin in, abdomen flattened and pelvis forward. Test your posture by standing with the head, back and buttocks against a wall and with feet about 4 inches from the wall. Push the low back hard against the wall. This is also an exercise.

f. Use comfortable shoes; avoid high heels. High heels tend to strain the back.

g. In sitting, keep feet firmly on the floor. The knees should be slightly higher than the hips. The front edge of the seat should not cut into the back of the thighs. The back of the chair should give support to the low back. Sit close to the desk. The back of the forearms should just rest on the desk surface without the body having to bend forward or the shoulders being raised.

h. The driver's seat in a car should be adjusted forward or backward to that the driver does not have stretch forward to reach the steering wheel or floor pedals (accelerator, clutch, brake). As with sitting in a chair, the low back needs adequate support. To help accomplish this, there are pads available which help give necessary support (Sacro-ease® is one)

i. Since ¼ to ⅓ of one daily time is spent in bed, posture there is important. The mattress should be firm, since the heavier parts of the body (hips and thighs) sink down, causing bad alignment and strain on the back when the bed is too soft. Putting a board under the mattress helps avoid this. An "egg crate" pad on a board may be the best.

3. Treatment of Acute Back Pain

a. Bed rest; firm mattress (see i. above); assume comfortable body position.

b. Ice massage (p. 60) several times daily.

c. Place a chair on floor and lie on your back, letting lower legs rest on seat of chair.

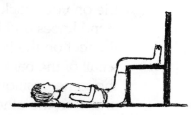

d. Warm tub bath (p. 34)
e. Acute back pain that does not yield to simple treatment should be evaluated by a physician. X-rays may be necessary.
f. After the symptoms have improved, treat as chronic back pain. Apply the principles listed under heading "Avoiding Straining the Back" (p. 88, # 2)

4. Treatment of Chronic Back Pain
   a. Continue to apply the principles given above - "Avoid Straining the Back" (p. 88, # 2)
   b. Exercise
      (1) A simple exercise consists of getting into a squatting position and holding the back of a chair for 3-5 minutes several times a day.

      Another is to lean forward while seated and to place one's head between the knees for several minutes and pull down back of head with hands. Also do exercise described in 3-c above.

(2) Lie on your back on the floor. Bend knees and hips. Keeping the feet on the floor, push the small of the back into the floor. In the same position, bend one knee and then the other, touching the knee to the chin using hands and arms to pull each leg up.

(3) Walking is good exercise for the back. Choose a flat level course. Assume proper posture as described above. Gradually increase distance.

(4) Stiffness of joints and bands of tissue across them (fascia) is an important part of poor posture and back pain. Such back pain may be associated with menstrual cramps. Refer to the section on treatment of this problem; the exercises described there will be beneficial here also (p. 138).

II. Nervous Disorders

A. Stress

  1. Definition—"An intense force, strain, agent or mental condition which produces a defense reaction. This reaction may be physiological or within normal limits and harmless, but if continued or intensified may lead to pathological lesions." *Taber's Cyclopedic Medical Dictionary*, p. 1377. Ed. 14.

     "Stress is the spice of life. it is associated with every type of activity. All of the systems of the body operate in a framework of exercise and movement, laws of life. Activity produces stress— which is basically essential to health. Who would enjoy a life of 'no hits, no runs, no errors'? The western world is racked by the insatiable demand for less work and more pay, yet the fatal enemy of all utopias is boredom." *Selye*, 1974.

  2. Types of Stress—Hans Selye, a Canadian endocrinologist, defines stress as the non-specific response of the body to any demand made on it. Let's illustrate it this way: Suppose you are driving down the highway with some urgency (about 70 m.p.h. of urgency), and you happen to glance in the rearview mirror. You see a familiar black and white automobile. Then the very thing you feared happens - the officer

flicks on his red light. You experience what we might call situational stress. *Selye*, 1974.

The businessman who is under constant pressure from his clients and employees alike, the air-traffic controller who knows that a moment of distraction may mean death to hundreds of people, the athlete who desperately wants to win a race, and the husband who helplessly watches his wife slowly and painfully dying of cancer—all suffer from stress. In spite of variations in the types of stress, the body responds in a rather stereotyped manner. Selye, 1974.

Our illustration of the officer's red light is an example of acute, or immediate, stress. The incoming information relays a message to the brain, the brain turns up the sympathetic nerve system, which in turn triggers the adrenal glands to release two chemical messengers, hormones called epinephrine and norepinephrine. These chemicals tune up the chemistry of the cells to the level of the emergency and several reactions take place. The lids and pupils of the eyes tend to open up. The peripheral blood vessels constrict, the heart rate increases, and the vessels of the heart enlarge. The lungs are called into action. The rate and depth of breathing are increased. The blood vessels inside the muscles open to supply them with more oxygen and fuel. *Baldwin*, 1972.

3. Vehicles of Stress—But what about the businessman under constant pressure? This can be termed chronic, or long-term stress. He is liable to develop high blood pressure, stomach ulcers, inflammation of the colon. Stress may aggravate his arthritis, contribute to chronic fatigue, insomnia, and headache. *Baldwin*, 1972.

There are other significant sources of stress. What about working with a bear? Or living with one! We might call the first occupational stress, and the latter home stress. Perhaps one reason why so many homes "break up" in our modern culture is because family members vent their pent-up frustrations of the day on each other at home, when they "Let their hair down." *Baldwin*, 1972.

Some vehicles of stress are products of the fast pace of modern living. For thousands of years, human beings traveled at a maximum of 15 - 20 miles per hour—and that for very short distances. During the past 75 years, speed of travel has increased to over 500 m.p.h. on land, 2,500 m.p.h. in air, and to speeds in excess of 25,000 m.p.h. in space. Communications technology has advanced to where we are now bombarded on the average with 560 advertisements, 10,000 to 20,000 words in print, several hours of T.V., and about 75 minutes of radio—all in single day. Not only that, but people under stress are often sources of stress as well.

4. How to Avoid Harmful Stress—One of the best ways to relieve undue stress is to engage in activities that release tension, such as physical exercise for those in sedentary patterns of life. One author declares that without exercise, the mind cannot be kept in working order. *My Life Today*, p. 130.

It is a little late to choose our parents or grandparents, and for most of us, the formative years are past. What, then, can we do about our stressful environment? Let's look at a few ways we can handle stress.

Living in a rural or semi-rural setting is helpful, even if one must travel several miles to work. Job satisfaction is a major factor. George Bernard Shaw gave this definition: "Labor is doing what we must; leisure is doing what we like." One man's work is another man's leisure. It is not a question of avoiding stress, but rather balancing healthy stress elements with others. Disagreeable tasks can even become challenges that bring satisfaction when solutions result from grappling with them.

Many of the most imminent men and women of history lived a long, happy life filled with challenges, many of them frustration and anxiety-producing at times. Consider people like Albert Schweitzer, Marian Anderson, Abraham Lincoln, Henry Ford, Tom Dooley, Thomas Edison, Marie Curie, and a host of others. Whether their lives were long or short, they responded optimistically to the challenges. *Selye*, 1974.

What can we do with stressful circumstances over which we have no control? Remember the prayer attributed to St Francis of Assisi: "Lord grant me the serenity to accept the things I cannot change, the courage to change the things I can, and the wisdom to know the difference." The ability to adapt, to be empathetic and understanding—how much we need these characteristics these days! It would be safe to say that 90% of all the causes of unhealthy stress would be eliminated, if everyone, individually and corporately, began to practice The Golden Rule. Wouldn't it be better to strike at the root of the problem, instead of just treating the symptoms? The Good Book says that stress factors will increase to the point where men's hearts will fail them for fear because of the things coming upon the world. Luke 2:26.

It is reassuring that there is superhuman help available. Under inspiration, John the Apostle wrote: "Perfect love casts out fear." The Divine Comforter assures us: "I will never leave thee nor forsake thee." Peter urges us to: "Cast every worry you have upon Him,… He takes care of you." I John 4:18; Hebrews 13:5; I Peter 5:7.

Who needs stress? We all do! But stress can be controlled, both by balancing stress factors with compensation activities, and by avoiding or modifying harmful stress elements in your life. The results will mean a happier life, that will serve to benefit and encourage others.

5. Simple Treatments That are Helpful—Most stress is manifested in muscle tension. The following simple water treatments enhance muscle relaxation:

   a. Fomentations to the spine (p. 6).
   b. Home Russian Bath: 15-20 minutes (p. 26).
   c. Neutral tub bath (p. 34).
   d. Hot and cold shower: relief of fatigue (p. 51).
   e. Hot foot bath (p. 1).
   f. Hot tub bath: relief of fatigue (p. 30).

g. Massage

B. Anxiety

    1. Description—This is a concern respecting some event, future or uncertain, which disturbs the mind and keeps it in a state of painful uneasiness accompanied by a distressing sense of pressure in the vicinity of the heart (Webster). There is an associated emotional disturbance, nervous tension, mental fatigue, and psychosomatic (functional) symptoms involving the autonomic nervous system. The psychosomatic symptoms may actually lead to serious disease involving high blood pressure, stroke, heart disease, etc. The best way to manage anxiety is trust in Divine grace. There follows a series of quotations from E. G. White regarding anxiety.

"God does not condemn prudence and foresight in the use of the things of this life, but the feverish care, the undue anxiety, with respect to worldly things is not in accordance with His will." *Counsels on Stewardship*, p. 159

"Because God's love is so great and so unfailing, the sick should be encouraged to trust in Him and be cheerful. To be anxious about themselves tends to cause weakness and disease. If they will rise above depression and gloom, their

prospect of recovery will be better...."
Ministry of Healing, P. 229.

"That which brings sickness of body and mind to nearly all is dissatisfied feelings and discontented repinings. They have not God, they have not the hope which reaches to that within the veil, which is as an anchor to the soul both sure and steadfast. All who possess this hope will purify themselves even as He is pure. Such are free from restless longings, repinings, and discontent; they are not continually looking for evil and brooding over borrowed trouble. But we see many who are having a time of trouble beforehand; anxiety is tamped upon every feature; they seem to find no consolation, but have a continual fearful looking for some dreadful evil. Such dishonor God, and bring the religion of Christ into disrepute. They have not true love for God, nor for their companions and children. Their affections have become morbid. But vain amusements will never correct the minds of such. They need the transforming influence of the Spirit of God in order to be happy. They need the transforming influence of the Spirit of God in order to be happy. They need to be benefitted by the mediation of Christ, in order to realize

consolation, divine and substantial."
Testimonies, Vol. 1, p. 566.

"No tears are shed that God does not
notice. There is no smile that he does
not mark. if we would but fully believe
this, all undue anxieties would be
dismissed." *Steps to Christ*, p. 86

"Jesus is our friend; all heaven is
interested in our welfare. We should not
allow the perplexities and worries of
everyday life to fret the mind and cloud
the brow. If we do, we shall always have
something to vex and annoy. We should
not indulge a solicitude that only frets
and wears us, but does not help us to
bear trials." *Steps to Christ*, p. 121-122.

"You need not weary yourself with busy
anxieties and needless cares. Work on
for the day, faithfully doing the work
which God's providence assigns you,
and he will have a care for you. Jesus
will deepen and widen your blessings."
Testimonies, Vol II, p. 576.

"In trusting in God continually there is
safety, there will not be a constant fear
of future evil. This borrowed care and
anxiety will cease. We have a heavenly
Father who careth for His children, and
will and does make His grace sufficient
in every time of need. When we take
into our own hands the management of

the things that concern us, and depend upon our own wisdom for success, we may well have anxiety and anticipate danger and loss, for it will most certainly come upon us." *Testimonies*, Vol. II, p. 72.

   3. As already indicated, anxiety leads to other problems. We shall next discuss nervous tension, headache, and lack of sleep (insomnia).

C. Nervous Tension

   1. Description—Nervous tension is a major cause of disease today. By its influence on nerves, glands, organs and blood vessels, it can produce peptic ulcer, high blood pressure, colitis, and possibly asthma and arthritis, as well as many other disorders and disabilities. There is no one cause for tension, so its treatment must include a number of factors.

   2. Treatment

     a. Alcohol, tobacco, tea, coffee, and cola drinks all contain substances which irritate the nerves. Avoid them ("A cup of tea made from catnip herb will quiet the nerves" *Selected Messages*, Vol II, p. 297)

     b. Certain vitamins (C and B complex) and minerals (calcium, potassium, phosphorus, magnesium) are needed by nerves and muscles. The diet should contain ample quantities of food rich in these elements. Such foods are fresh fruits, vegetables, nuts and seeds, whole grains and cereals. Stop intake of refined foods, excessive starches, sugars and fats.

c. Avoid vinegar, baking soda, pepper, spices and excessive salt.

d. Shallow breathing decreases oxygen intake to which nerve function is especially sensitive. Practice deep abdominal breathing exercises for calming nerves and inducing sleep.

e. Top authorities are agreed that exercise is the best sedative and tranquilizer. It is a vital remedy for tension and many conditions secondary to tension. Give it a good try. Walking and gardening are two of the best exercises to start with.

f. Get adequate rest. Some need nine or ten hours sleep at night; some need a nap during the day.

g. Avoid excitement of all kinds—arguments, anger, watching movies and television, reading novels, etc.

h. Avoid stimulants, sedatives, pain killers, and tranquilizers which do not cure, which may be habit-forming, and which may put an added stress on the nerves.

i. Use warm and cold showers (p. 40), neutral tub baths at night (p. 34), cold mitten friction (p. 17) in the mornings, and other water treatments to relax and tone up the system. Use these measures instead of drugs.

j. Fear, perplexity, mental anguish and depression are major causes of tension and exhaustion. The best remedy is an unwavering trust in God and His loving care for you, which can be gained by study of the promises in His Word, by prayer, and by daily submission to His will. Peace and serenity can thus be developed which will enable one to endure great difficulties. Develop, also, positive mental traits such as cheerfulness, thankfulness and thoughtfulness of others.

Precautions: An abrupt personality change may be organic in nature, as for example, that caused by a brain tumor. Some patients who appear to show only nervous tension at first will begin to show bizarre mental and emotional symptoms or suicidal tendencies suggestive of serious mental disease later on. Such patients should be seen by a psychiatrist.

D. Headache
   1. Description—Since most headaches are
      due to nervous tension, they are
      included in this section. Severe tension
      headaches usually begin in the neck and
      back of the head; surprisingly, they often
      awaken one from sleep or start just after
      one arises. They may or may not be
      associated with nausea and are
      characterized by a steady ache.

      True migraine headaches are unilateral,
      usually behind one eye.. There is often
      blurred vision or spots before the eyes.
      They rapidly build up to an intense,
      throbbing pain, often with severe nausea
      and vomiting, and are usually recurrent.
   2. Treatment:
      a. Hot half-bath in tub (p. 53), sitting
         with legs covered with water. Have
         water as hot as tolerated, with one
         table spoon of mustard added. Cold
         compress to the head (p. 22); end
         with cold rub or pail pour.
      b. Skip a meal, drink one to two quarts
         of bitter hop; go to bed in a quiet,
         dark room.
      c. For migraine:
         (1) Take a warm, saline enema.
         (2) Use above measures.
         (3) Lie in bed, practicing slow, deep
             abdominal breathing at first sign
             of an impending attack. Ice bag

to head or put head under cold shower at beginning of attack, after #1 and #2 have been completed. Beware of drug dependence.

    d. For tension headaches: try warm fomentations (p. 6) to back and neck, ice pack to back of head with hot foot bath (p. 62 & 1). Massage of back, shoulders, and neck, with special attention to any tender areas.

  3. Precautions—Headaches may be due to many organic causes—from eye strain to high blood pressure to brain tumor. Abrupt onset of headache in a previously well person, localized pain. visual disturbances (except in migraine headache), neurological signs or symptoms, changes in pain with position change, and change in headache pattern—these are all danger signals.

E. Insomnia

  1. Description—Although not a disease, this can be a distressing symptom to many tense and nervous people and may lead to drug dependency or habituation.

  2. Hydrotherapy:

    a. Neutral bath or shower (p. 34)

    b. Wet sheet pack (p. 42)

    c. Massage

    d. Fomentations to the spine (p. 6)

    e. Home Russian Bath for 15 - 20 minutes (p. 26)

    f. Hot Foot Bath (p. 1)

    g. Hot mitten friction (p. 19)

3. Herbs:

    a. Hop tea (very bitter - lemon juice helps). Prepare one to two quarts to drink at bedtime and during the night. ("Hop tea will induce sleep." Selected Messages, Vol. II, p. 297).

    b. Catnip tea. Use at bedtime and during night, as needed.

4. Many find it helpful to drink water early in the day and to drink nothing within one hour of bedtime.

5. Deep breathing exercises. Adequate fresh air in the room. Make sure you are warm.

6. Lying down for a few minutes several times during the day may help break the tension.

7. Take long walks and other exercise daily to produce physical fatigue—"the best sedative and tranquilizer."

8. Avoid tea, coffee, late and heavy suppers, rich and spicy foods, excitement, and sleeping pills (they may actually decrease one's ability to sleep naturally.).

9. Listen to soft, relaxing music or read inspirational (not exciting) materials.

10. A soft blinder to obliterate all light is often helpful.

11. See last suggestion under "Nervous
Tension" above.

III. Skin Problems

A. Lymphangitis ("Blood Poison")

    1. Definition—inflammation of lymph vessels. It is characterized by a red streak passing upward, usually from a local infection site. There is usually a fever. There is also usually swelling of lymph nodes as, for example, in the arm pit. Bacteria (usually streptococci) are being encountered by the white blood cells in a homeostatic attempt of the body to prevent generalized invasion of the blood stream (septicemia). This is a dangerous condition.

    With the use of antibiotics, treatment is much more effective now than before their availability. As an adjunct alternate, hot and cold local baths (p. 51). When given persistently will help in stimulating the defense against the infection.

B. Boils and Abscesses

    1. Usually caused by infection due to staphylococcal infections. The dosage of germs, breaks in the skin, general hygiene, and body resistance play a part in determining who will fall victim to such infections. often the germs will be passed to other family members by careless handling of contaminated clothing. An infected person's clothing and bed linens should be handled very carefully and washed separately.

2. Treatment:
   a. Avoid all sweets, rich or greasy foods. Sugar decreases the white blood cells' ability to destroy germs. Eat foods rich in vitamins A and C (fresh fruits and vegetables).
   b. Local treatments:
      (1) Hot and cold local baths (p. 51) or compresses; give as hot as can be tolerated. Repeat every two to four hours in acute cases.
      (2) Poultices of Epsom salts or charcoal (p. 75)
      (3) Cleanse the area with warm water and soap.
   c. Build up general resistance—adequate rest, exercise, plenty of water, natural well-balanced diet, avoidance of stress.

C. Burns:

This discussion is for local first degree burns (First degree burns are only superficial).

Use cold until pain subsides, then use neutral temperature water until there is no pain when part is withdrawn from the water. Reason: if part is put in cold and then withdrawn, usually pain becomes more intense when part is withdrawn. With neutral following the cold, this is usually avoided. Apply aloe vera gel.

D. Pressure Sores:

Taking care of the chronically ill, debilitated, bedfast patient presents certain problems which are not so obvious. One of the problems is the danger of the development of pressure sores (decubitus ulcers). When a well person lies in such a position so that pressure on local skin area is threatening to damage the skin and deeper layers, he will change position even during sleep because of the discomfort. Thus, normally the area will again receive good blood supply. If, however, the patient lacks sensation in the area, or if he cannot move, or if general tissue nutrition is poor and he is debilitated, then the tissue that is being compressed may actually die. The result is a pressure sore. Pressure sores can be very deep and may seriously affect health. The most common site of such sores is over the sacrum (near the lower end of the spine).

Pressure sores should never be allowed to develop. The most important means to prevent them is to change the position of the body frequently—at least every 2 - 3 hours. Also, keep the skin dry, massage, alcohol rub, and alternate hot and cold will help. Frequent bathing for cleanliness is imperative.

IV. Respiratory Problems

A. The Common cold

   1. Definition—A true cold is a mild illness with little or no fever, and the symptoms are confined to the nose and throat, causing mucous membrane inflammation and congestion. There is an increase in the nasal secretion and often sneezing. Transmission to another is by droplets and by contact.

   2. Causes

      a. Exposure to the virus—It has been observed that isolated people do not catch colds as on an island (even though they may be chilled) until a ship comes in.

      b. Chilling—For people who are living in an environment where the virus is prevalent, then chilling disposes to getting sick.

      c. Impaired Immunity—Some individuals have a natural resistance to the common cold, whereas others repeatedly get sick.

      d. Stress—People that are stressed and overworked seem more disposed to catching cold.

      e. Diet—A good diet program seems to help in preventing the cold attack. Sugar and sweets should be avoided.

   3. Treatment:

      a. Fomentation to the chest and back (p. 6) in combination with the hot foot bath (p. 1), the cold compress to the head, and cold mitten friction (p. 17), or ice rub (p. 11, # 12), followed perhaps by the cold shower or cold tub bath (p. 37). Steam inhalation (p. 70) may also be used. The patient must drink adequate water with the treatment. Following the treatment he should rest so as to eliminate the added heat so he will not perspire in his clothing after dressing.

   b. For the best application one may employ the Home Russian Bath (p. 26) or the hot tub bath (p. 30).

   c. Throughout the day the patient should drink much water and fruit juices.

   d. Treatments should be given daily.

4. The patient should be careful not to expose others to the infection.

5. Complication—The common cold may be followed by secondary infection in the nose, sinuses, throat, larynx. bronchi or lungs.

6. Quotations pertaining to colds and respiratory problems from Ellen G. White:

   a. "I should do a very unwise thing to enter a cool room when in a perspiration; I should show myself an unwise steward to allow myself to sit in a draft, and thus expose myself so as to take cold. I should be unwise to sit with cold feet and limbs, and thus drive back the blood from the extremities to the brain or internal organs. I should always protect my feet in damp weather." *Counsels on Diet and Food*, p. 302.

b. "If the child has taken cold, it is generally owing to the wrong management of the mother. If she covers its head, as well as its body, while sleeping, in a short time it will be in a perspiration, caused by labored breathing, because of the lack of pure, vital air, When she takes it from beneath the covering, it is almost sure to take cold." *Selected Messages*, Vol II, p. 469.

c. "The arms being naked, exposes the infant to constant cold, and congestion of lung or brain. These exposures prepare the way for the infant to become sickly and dwarfed." *Selected Messages*, Vol. II, p. 469.

d. "When we overtax our strength, and become exhausted, we are liable to take cold, and at such times there is danger of disease assuming a dangerous form." *Testimonies*, Vol. III, p. 13.

e. "Most persons would receive benefit from a cool or tepid bath every day, morning or evening, Instead of increasing the liability to take cold, a bath, properly taken, fortifies against cold, because it improves the circulation...." *Ministry of Healing*, p. 276.

f. "The dress should fit easily, obstructing neither the circulation of the blood or a free, full, natural respiration. The feet should be suitably protected from cold and damp. Clad in this way, we can take exercise in the open air, even in the dew of morning and evening, or after a fall or rain or snow, without fear of taking cold." *Child Guidance*, p. 425.

g. "...no one can have good digestive powers and a clear brain who will eat largely of sweet cookies and cream cake and all kinds of pies, and partake of a great variety of food at one meal. When we do this, and then take cold, the whole system is so clogged and enfeebled that it has no power of resistance, no strength to combat disease." *Counsels on Diet and Food*, p. 334.

h. "Those who have excluded the air from their sleeping rooms, should begin to change their course immediately. They should let in air by degrees, and increase its circulation until they can bear it winter and summer, with no danger of taking cold." *Counsels on Health*, p. 57, 58.

i. "The sickroom, if possible, should have a draft of air through it, day and night. The draft should not come directly upon the invalid while burning fevers are raging; there is but little danger of taking cold." *Counsels on Health*, p. 56.

j. "The electric power of the brain, promoted by mental activity, vitalizes the whole system, and is thus an invaluable aid to resisting disease." *Education*, p. 197.

k. "Imagination is active; they expect to take cold, and they will have it." *Counsels on Health*, p. 97.

l. "Bring to your aid the power of the will, which will resist cold, and will give energy to the nervous system." *Counsels on Health*, p. 54.

m. "Morning exercise, in walking in the free, invigorating air of heaven…is the surest safeguard against cold, coughs, congestion of the brain and lungs…and an hundred other diseases." *Healthful Living*, p. 210.

n. "Drug takers are never well, They are always taking cold, which causes extreme suffering, because of the poison all through their systems." *Healthful Living*, p. 209.

B. Sinusitis
   1. Description—The acute form is due to
      infection of the mucous membrane
      lining of the sinuses by either viral or
      bacterial agents, and is almost always
      concomitant with, or a complication of,
      other respiratory diseases. It may
      produce blockage of the natural sinus
      passages with accumulation of fluid or
      pus in the sinus, severe pain, and high
      fever. The chronic form is often due to
      indolent infection from inadequately
      treated acute sinusitis. However, other
      factors such as allergies and sinus or
      nasal polyps often complicate the
      picture. For this reason, medical advice
      should be sought in cases of
      slow-resolving or recurrent sinusitis.
   2. Treatment (Acute Phase)
      a. General measures (see Acute
         Bronchitis, p. 123)
      b. Hydrotherapy (as often as necessary)
         (1) Alternate hot and cold to the face
             (p. 51)
         (2) Fomentation to the face (p. 6)
         (3) Heat lamp or infrared to the face
         (4) Alternating hot and cold showers
      c. Steam inhalations with a few drops
         of pine and eucalyptus oil in the
         water (p. 70).
   3. Precautions: Unremitting, severe, or
      increasing pain or headache, or high
      fever of more than a few hours

duration—failure of these symptoms to respond to the preceding measures is usually indicative of the presence of sinus blockage. The doctor may need to drain the sinuses and prescribe antibiotics, although early and vigorous treatment often makes this unnecessary.

C. Sore Throat (Pharyngitis)

1. Description—Most of the time sore throat is viral in origin and merely accompanies other respiratory illnesses, It may, however, be caused by bacteria such as the streptococcus which is potentially serious and should, thus, have immediately medical attention. Usually the "scratch" or "burning" sore throat, accompanied by a cold and with very little fever, can be treated conservatively for at least twenty-four hours.

2. Treatment:
   a. Gargles—alternating with hot salt water, as hot as tolerated, and cold charcoal water, one tablet to a glass—every few hours.
   b. Hydrotherapy:
      (1) Alternating hot and cold packs to the neck (p. 51)
      (2) Alternating hot and cold showers
      (3) Heating compress to throat overnight (p. 65)
      (4) Steam inhalation (p. 70)

D. Ear Ache (Otitis media)
   1. Description—Earache is, again, as
      symptom indication infection by either
      viruses or bacteria of the tissues of the
      ear canal outside the eardrum (otitis
      external), or behind the ear drum (otitis
      media). Both conditions usually
      complicate other ailments, but they can
      also be primary, Otitis media is the more
      serious, since swelling or pus can build
      up pressure behind the drum, causing it
      to rupture, perhaps with permanent
      damage to the hearing; or what is worse,
      the infection may spread to the inner ear
      and then to the brain to cause
      meningitis. Mastoiditis or chronic
      draining otitis are also complications
      which may occur.

      Therefore, in view of the seriousness of
      the complication which may accompany
      an earache, *a doctor should be called
      immediately* to make an accurate
      diagnosis and to institute prompt
      treatment. Measures noted below should
      be used only while awaiting a doctor, or
      in the event of the unavailability of a
      doctor. They may also be used after the
      doctor's visit, but only with his approval.
   2. Treatment:
      a. After checking with the doctor,
         institute general measures as below

b. Hydrotherapy:
   (1) Hot foot bath with one
        tablespoon of mustard;
        fomentations extending from one
        ear across throat to other
        ear—occasionally remove and
        rub with ice water and dry.
   (2) Hot bath, cold pour, vigorous rub
        with fomentation, as above.
   (3) Drops of warm olive oil in ear
        only on approval of doctor (as oil
        can obstruct his vision of the
        drum), heating pad, hot water
        bottle, heat lamp, simultaneous
        application of hot water bottle to
        one ear and cold water bottle to
        the other ear (alternate these).
   (4) In the case of small children,
        heating compress (p. 65) to the
        feet and lower legs has been
        found very helpful.
3. Precautions—As noted above, progress
    should be followed closely by the doctor
    until pain and fever are gone. Antibiotics
    and surgical lancing of the eardrum may
    be necessary.
E. Acute Laryngitis
   1. Definition—Acute Laryngitis is acute
       inflammation of the voice box and vocal
       cords, characterized by hoarseness or
       ability only to whisper as well as
       difficulty in swallowing.

2. Causes:
    a. Improper use of the voice
    b. Exposure to cold and wet
    c. Extension of infection from the nose
       and throat or common cold
    d. Inhalation of noxious vapors or dust
    e. Allergy
3. Treatment
    a. Complete rest of voice (no singing)
    b. Steam inhalation (p. 70) at least for
       15 minutes (every 2-3 hours for 2
       days)
    c. Heating compress to throat (p. 65)
    d. Adequate water drinking
    e. Sweating treatment such as Home
       Russian Bath (p. 26)

F. Chronic Laryngitis
    1. Definition—recurring or persistent
       inflammation of the voice box. It is
       characterized by hoarseness, tickling in
       the throat, and cough.
    2. Causes—Often follows acute laryngitis
       and may be secondary to infection in the
       throat, nose or sinuses. Improper use of
       the voice or smoking may be causes.
       Alcohol drinking may also be a cause.
       The symptoms of chronic laryngitis may
       indicate the presence of cancer of the
       larynx.
    3. Treatment:
        a. Discontinue smoking or use of
           alcohol.

b. Correct other problems in the nose and throat.
c. Minimize use of the voice. Learn to place the voice properly (see quotations from Ellen G. White below).
d. Steam inhalations (p. 70)
e. Heating throat compresses (p. 65)
f. General tonic treatments such as cold mitten friction (p. 17)
g. Consult nose and throat medical specialist.

4. Quotations from Ellen G. White:

"Voice culture is a subject that has much to do with the health of students. The youth should be taught how to breathe properly, and how to read in such a way that no unnatural strain shall come on the throat and lungs, but that the work shall be shared by the abdominal muscles. Speaking from the throat, letting the sound come from the upper part of the vocal organs, impairs the health of these organs and decreases their efficiency. The abdominal muscles are to do the heaviest part of the labor, the throat being used as the channel. Many have died who might have lived had they been taught how to use the voice correctly. The right use of the abdominal muscles in reading and speaking will prove a remedy for many voice and chest difficulties, and the means of prolonging life." *Counsels to Teachers*, p. 297.

"Speaking from the throat, letting the words come out from the upper extremity of the vocal organs, all the time fretting and irritating them, is not the best way to preserve health or to increase the efficiency of those organs. You should take a full inspiration and let the action come from the abdominal muscles. Let the lungs be only the channel, but do not depend upon them to do the work. If you let your words come from deep down, exercising the abdominal muscles, you can speak to thousands with just as much ease as you can speak to ten." *Testimonies*, Vol. II p. 616.

G. Acute Bronchitis
  1. Description—An infection or inflammation of the bronchial tubes by either viruses or bacteria. It frequently accompanies, or is a complication of, other respiratory illnesses. The cardinal symptom is cough which may or may not be productive of sputum. Wheezing may be present, along with chest tightness and dull ache which occurs diffusely throughout the chest. There is usually moderate fever.

123

2. Treatment:
    a. General measures (see below).
    b. Hydrotherapy:
        (1) Hot bath at bedtime for 6 - 10 minutes followed by neutral bath for 20 minutes (p. 30 & 34)
        (2) Fomentation to chest every 2 hours, followed by heating compress—carefully avoid exposure of back of neck, chest or shoulders to draft or chill during treatment (p. 6).
        (3) Drink plenty of water—6-8 glasses daily
    c. General Measures:
        (1) Stay away from work and from other people. These conditions are mostly highly contagious and are thus easily transmitted to others.
        (2) Stay in bed during the fever stage. This will give the body's natural defense mechanisms their best chance of working efficiently.
        (3) Make sure the sick room is adequately ventilated with fresh air, neither too hot nor too cold. The temperature should actually be around 68°, which tends toward the cool side.
        (4) A fruit diet during the acute phase is most beneficial, especially if it is high in citrus

fruits. This provides extra vitamin C which most clinicians feel is helpful, even though excessive quantities of vitamin C have not been proven, in well-controlled studies, to shorten the course of respiratory disease. Some recommend a liquid diet of fruit juices. We feel that the whole-fruit diet is superior nutritionally and physiologically and is usually more acceptable to the patient. Hot, unsweetened lemonade is often soothing, however, and may be used freely.

(5) Avoid sweets and sugars of all kinds! There is abundant evidence that sugar interferes with the body's natural defense mechanisms and actually promotes the growth of disease-causing organism.

(6) Short walks outside, as soon as the fever is over, with proper clothing protection, will help promote the return of strength and a feeling of well-being.

(7) The use of certain herb teas can be pleasant, symptomatically helpful, and harmless, having no side effects as do powerful drugs.

(8) Steam vaporizer at bedside constantly. Steam inhalations may be helpful (p. 70).

(9) Honey-eucalyptus cough syrup (few drops of oil of eucalyptus to a cup of honey) as needed.

3. Precautions—High or prolonged fever, failure to improve in thirty-six to forty-eight hours, increasing symptoms or prostration, bloody sputum, shortness of breath, or pleurisy—all suggest serious complications and require prompt medical intervention.

H. Chronic Bronchitis

1. Description—cough of prolonged duration (more than two weeks). Fever is usually negligible or low-grade. There are often complication factors such as asthma, allergies, or smoking. Since a chronic cough is non-specific and may be caused by many things in addition to bronchitis, such as emphysema, tuberculosis, or lung cancer, all patients should be seen first by a doctor for accurate diagnosis. Only afterward, with the doctor's permission, should the following measures be tried.

2. Treatment:

a. Follow a program similar to that given for acute bronchitis, except treat less vigorously; give hydrotherapy less frequently.

Program to build up general resistance:
- (1) Simple, nourishing diet
- (2) Avoid exposure to wet or cold
- (3) Keep extremities well-clothed
- (4) Out-of-doors life

I. Atelectasis (Collapsed Lung)

Taking care of the chronically ill, debilitated patient presents certain problems which are not so obvious. One of these is a collapse (atelectasis) of a large portion of the lung. Such a collapse decreases breathing ability and furthermore sets the stage for infection.

It is well to understand the mechanism. The debilitated patient may have an incidental cold or other condition leading to mucus formation in the bronchial tubes. Because of his debilitated state, he may lack the desire or strength to cough up the mucus. The mucus may collect in the bronchial tube to form a plug. When that happens, the part of the lung which is ventilated through that bronchus is completely closed off—the air there is trapped. Now this trapped air becomes absorbed by the blood and consequently that part of the lung collapses. If the lung tissue involved is large, then breathing may become difficult, but usually the more serious situation is that the lung tissue which has collapsed is prone to develop infection, possibly pneumonia.

Now, if measures are taken to move the plug out, the atelectasis would be prevented. This can be done either by causing the patient to move the chest by the application of sudden cold or by assisting the patient to cough by pressing on the chest. The patient could be given some device to blow into. Fomentations to the chest, alternated with very cold cloth, may be employed (p. 6).

J. Influenza
  1. Description—A viral condition known as influenza usually occurs in epidemic form, thus making diagnosis more certain. Symptoms may be similar to those of a common cold, but with higher fever, often up to 103°-104° in adults, frequently accompanied by prostration. A characteristic symptom is severe aching of the whole body. Certain specific viral strains, such as Asian or Hong Kong Flu, may cause other symptoms peculiar to that particular variety. These are usually self-limited in about a week's time, but are often followed by persistent nagging symptoms and prolonged weakness.
  2. Treatment:
    a. All of the general measures (see p. 123, Acute Bronchitis), with emphasis on bed rest.

b. Hydrotherapy (one or more treatments, two to four times daily):
   (1) Home steam bath with hot foot bath and cold to head until sweating profusely. Wrap in blanket and put to bed immediately. Hot lemonade in abundance. NOTE: After profuse sweating, temperature usually drops 1°-2°.
   (2) Hot immersion bath followed by cold mitten friction or cold towel rub twice daily (p. 17).
   (3) Copious water drinking.
   (4) Keep warm, rest in bed.
   (5) Hot blanket pack (p. 42).
   (6) Fomentations to chest (p. 6), cold mitten friction (p. 17), hot foot bath (p. 1)—for cough.
3. Precautions—same as in common colds (p. 112), except that fever will be higher in flu, and chills are common early in course of illness. Convalescence will be more prolonged, and the patient should not be around others until completely afebrile[*] for at least twenty-four hours.

---

[*] Normal temperature (no fever)

V. Digestion Disorders
A. Dyspepsia. "Indigestion" or "Acid Stomach"
   1. Description—symptoms of discomfort often occurring after eating. The burping, burning sensation in the epigastrium, bloating, and "indigestion" is often due to nervous tension and to wrong eating habits such as eating too fast, eating too much, eating between meals, eating the wrong kinds and combinations of foods, and partaking of excessive spices. It may be caused or aggravated by coffee, tea, smoking or alcohol.
   2. Treatment:
      a. Avoid rich, fried, greasy, spicy foods. Eat only at regular times, at least five hours apart. Avoid eating a heavy meal in the evening. Avoid any food that definitely causes irritation. Do not eat a wide variety of foods at any one meal.
      b. Discard coffee, tea, other caffeine drinks, alcohol and tobacco.
      c. Relaxing outdoor exercise such as walking or gardening.
      d. Take two charcoal tablets as needed for distress. Use ripe olives at mealtimes.
      e. Drink plenty of water between meals, but not with meals. Slippery elm or catnip tea may be helpful.

      f. Hydrotherapy
        (1) Fomentations to the upper abdomen (p. 6)
        (2) Neutral tub bath at bedtime (p. 34)
      g. Follow suggestions in section on "Nervous Tension," (p. 102).
    3. Precautions—Since these symptoms may be mimicked exactly by peptic ulcer or by more serious diseases, persistent or frequently recurring symptoms deserve medical attention for possible x-ray and other studies.

B. Diarrhea
    1. Description—a symptom of many conditions of the colon. It is associated most commonly with viral infections, injudicious eating, or "food poisoning." The latter, which may cause acute nausea, vomiting, and diarrhea within hours after eating, is due to contamination of food with the staphylococcal germ, a toxin is produced which causes the symptoms. It is often relatively mild and self-limited, may be prostrating.
    2. Treatment:
      a. Limit diet to bananas, white potatoes, rice, scraped apple, boiled milk. Avoid coarse and laxative foods during acute-symptom stage.
      b. Bed rest if acute.

        c. A cold pack to the lower abdomen may be helpful.

        d. Charcoal tablets, one to twelve every four hours until controlled (p. 75).

        e. One rounded tablespoonful of carob in a glass of boiled milk three times daily.

    3. Precautions—Fever is indicative of (1) bacterial infection, as with salmonella organism, (2) diverticulitis, or (3) other serious disorders. Cramping may accompany any diarrhea, but rapidly subsides in the benign forms. Watch out for severe or prolonged pain, recurrent diarrhea, or any diarrhea not clearing in twenty-four hours. Call then for medical aid.

C. Constipation

    1. Description—Simple constipation is due to eating too many refined foods which are low in bulk and roughage, to lack of exercise, to an inadequate intake of water, and often to the taking of constipating medications, as well as to lack of regular bowel habits.

    2. Treatment:

        a. Use bulky, natural foods freely, such as prunes, dried figs, oranges, apples, raw vegetables, whole-wheat bread and cereals. Avoid excessive milk.

b. Avoid refined sugars, starches and rich or greasy foods. Eat nuts sparingly.

c. Drink at least eight glasses of water a day—two upon arising, two between breakfast and lunch, two between lunch and supper, and two at bedtime.

d. Take one ounce of Torumel yeast or rice polishings in water daily. Use ripe olives with each meal.

e. Get plenty of outdoor exercise and adequate rest.

f. Have a regular time for elimination.

g. Flaxseed tea at night, and a glass of hot water and prune juice on arising may be helpful.

h. Deep breathing exercises.

i. Hydrotherapy:
   (1) Fomentation and cold rub (p. 6) to abdomen
   (2) Graduated enemas if necessary—less and cooler daily.

3. Precaution—Any abrupt change in bowel habits is a danger signal and should be investigated medically. Otherwise, observe general precaution.

D. Nausea and Vomiting

1. Description—The only types of nausea and vomiting that should be treated at home are (1) the acute form related to viral infection ("intestinal flu"), (2) simple upset stomach often from injudicious

eating or "food poisoning," or (3) that
related to migraine headache. The first is
often epidemic and associated with
respiratory symptoms. The others can
usually be diagnosed early by history.

2. Treatment:
   a. Bed rest.
   b. Nothing by mouth until acute
      vomiting is over; then start with sips
      of peppermint tea. Seven-up® over
      cracked ice is often effective in
      children as well as adults.
   c. Give activated charcoal, 2 tablets
      ever 2-3 hours.
   d. Drink hot broth and juices; eat light
      diet and ripe olives.
   e. Hydrotherapy:
      (1) Ice bag to the upper abdomen
          (p. 62).
      (2) Some have success at times with
          fomentation to the abdomen (p. 6).
      (3) Precaution—Nausea and
          vomiting can be symptoms of
          almost any serious condition
          involving the internal organs, so if
          the condition does not clear
          promptly or if it recurs, one
          should call a doctor promptly.
          Vomiting from any cause,
          including psychogenic, may lead
          to serious dehydration at any
          age, if it continues. Observe the
          general precautions.

VI. Miscellaneous Conditions
A. Conjunctivitis
1. Description—an inflammation or infection by a virus or bacteria of the inside of the eyelids and surface of the ball. It causes redness, enlarged and engorged blood vessels ("bloodshot eyes"), mild to moderate burning and irritation, and often an exudate that may plaster the eyelids shut in the morning.
2. Treatment:
   a. Avoid sugar and sweets.
   b. Local treatment:
      (1) Saline eyewash—1 teaspoon of salt to one pint of boiled water.
      (2) Charcoal eyewash—1-2 teaspoons of charcoal to a pint of boiled water. Let charcoal settle and use the fluid drained off the top.
      (3) Charcoal poultices at night (p. 75). (For use of charcoal for eyes, see Selected Messages, Vol. II, P. 297.
      (4) Hot and cold compresses (p. 51).
3. Precautions—Many of these conditions are quite contagious. Stay away from people. If no improvement is noted in twenty-four hours, see an eye specialist. Considerable pain, soreness of the orbit on pressure, blurring, or other visual disturbances are all danger signals which may indicate deeper-seated infection

such as iritis, or perhaps even acute glaucoma. See an eye specialist immediately.

B. Dysmenorrhea (Painful Menstruation)

1. Description—Primary dysmenorrhea over the last half century has been labelled by some women as the "curse" and by gynecologists as an "enigma." At various times its proposed causes have been attributed to mental, nutritional, emotional. environmental and hormonal causes.

It is well recognized that a young woman who has severe menstrual cramps to the point of being incapacitated may be able to deliver a baby by natural methods—indicating that labor was minimal distress compared to her menstrual period. This suggests that she does not have a low pain tolerance as has been attributed to the pain of dysmenorrhea.

The best theory yet is the endocrine theory—which has been proven many times by the consistent use of birth-controls pills—namely: dysmenorrhea is minimal where a consistent level of estrogen and progesterone is given to inhibit ovulation.

Sir William Osler, in one of his lectures, said: "Menstruation is the tears of a disappointed uterus," meaning, of course, that the whole menstrual function is geared to produce a pregnancy, and when this does not occur, the "nest" that has been prepared inside the womb to house the pregnancy is discarded. This can be done in two ways: (1) dripping away like melting ice and seeping through a small cervic which is not painful, and (2) by separating the whole "nest" rather precipitously so that it dams up the funnel-shaped entrance to the cervical canal and the woman now has to "deliver" this clot through a reluctant cervix, which causes painful uterine contractions and nausea.

Generally, any program of exercise that on a consistent basis stimulates circulation will diminish painful menses. Also, a diet that is rich in "seed elements" (Genesis 1:28, 29) will provide raw materials for the production of hormones. This in turn will prevent premature shedding of the endometrium, which would cause pain.

Regular and adequate rest and sleep periods are also important, since fatigue causes congestion generally and the normal congestion prior to menstruation is increased, producing more pain.

Here, too, dress is important...If the extremities are poorly clad or unclad in cold weather, pelvic congestion is physiologically increased, and likewise the pain.

2. Treatment:
   a. Generally keep warm
   b. Hot foot bath (p. 1)
   c. Hot tub bath (p. 30)
   d. Hot fomentations (to pelvis or lumbar region) (p. 6)
   e. Exercises for dysmenorrhea

   The objective of the exercise is to stretch the shortened fascial ligamentous bands which extend between the lower back and the anterior aspect of the pelvis and legs. The shortened fascial ligamentous bands may result in an increased pelvic tilt and in the impingement and irritation of the peripheral nerves as they pass through or near the fascia.

   The exercise should be continued over a period of time, even after relief has been obtained. The exercise should be performed 3 times on each side, 3 times daily.
   f. Procedure of the exercise:
      (1) Stand in good alignment, left side of body about distance of the bent elbow from wall, feet together, left forearm and palm against wall, elbow shoulder

FACIAL STRETCH—SIDE VIEW

FACIAL STRETCH—FRONT VIEW

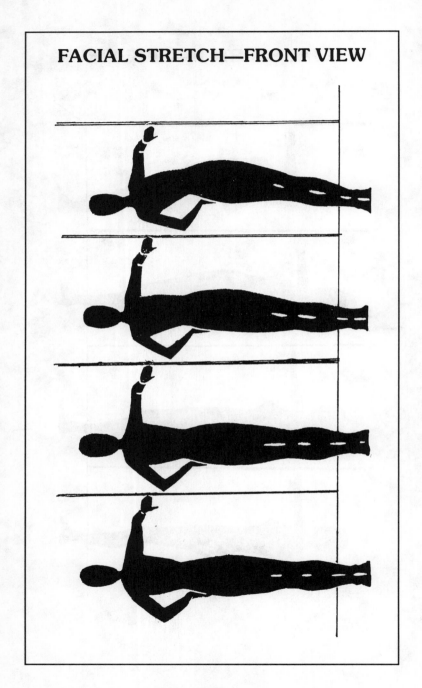

height, heel of right hand placed against posterior aspect of greater trochanter (hollow hip).

  (2) Contract abdominal and gluteal muscles strongly, tilting pelvis backward.

  (3) Slowly push hips forward and diagonally toward wall, applying pressure with hand.

  (4) Hold position.

  (5) Slowly return to starting position and repeat stretch 2 more times.

  (6) Repeat stretch 3 times on opposite side.

g. Things to remember:

  (1) Keep abdominal and gluteal muscles contracted strongly.

  (2) Keep knees extended.

  (3) Keep shoulders and elbow at right angle to wall, arm at shoulder height.

  (4) Keep shoulders relaxed and approximately over feet.

  (5) Keep elbow against wall and avoid twisting body.

  (6) Avoid touching wall with body.

  (7) Push hips diagonally forward to greatest possible extension.

(See pages 139 & 140 for illustrations.)

C. Phlebothrombosis (Venous Clotting)
   1. Taking care of the chronically ill,
      debilitated patient presents certain
      problems which are not so obvious. One
      of these problems is the development of
      a clot in the legs. The tendency for the
      patient to lie motionless results in a
      sluggish circulation. The pumping of the
      blood through the veins is stimulated by
      movement. Furthermore, there is
      constant pressure against the veins of the
      legs, especially the back of the lower legs
      (calves). This also slows the circulation.
      These factors, plus the general condition
      of the patient, favors clotting. Since
      there is not necessarily an inflammation,
      the clots do not become firmly attached.
      The clot might develop to a large
      length—even several inches. When such
      a clot is present, the condition is called
      phlebothrombosis (versus
      thrombophlebitis which is associated
      with an inflammation). Such a clot can
      easily be dislodged and travel up the
      large veins through the right side of the
      heart and then to the lungs. There, of
      course, it is stopped since it cannot pass
      through the lung capillaries. Such a large
      clot then will suddenly stop circulation
      and oxygenation. This will cause sudden
      death. Resuscitation is not possible. This
      is called pulmonary embolism.
      Pulmonary embolism used to be quite a

common occurrence when patients were confined to bed in a hospital and then, when they got up to leave the hospital, suddenly died.

The treatment of this situation is only PREVENTION. The formation of a clot can be prevented if the legs are moved frequently either by the patient or by an attendant. Even asking the patient to tighten his calf muscles frequently will help. Also, hydrotherapy and massage will help prevent clot formation.

The Chronically Ill Debilitated Bedfast Patient

Danger of:
1. Phlebothrombosis (p. 143)
2. Abnormal joint position and alignment (p. 87)
3. Lung atelectasis—pneumonia (p. 127 & 128)
4. Pressure sores (p. 111)

D. Fever
1. Description—Fever is always merely a symptom of disease, never an illness in itself. Small children may, however, develop high fevers of up to 104°-105° very rapidly, sometimes, apparently, in the absence of other symptoms. These

fevers are almost always due to the various respiratory viruses and are usually self-limited; the child often recovering almost as rapidly as the illness itself started. Prompt treatment may shorten the illness, provide symptomatic relief, and help to prevent complication.

2. Treatment:
   a. Warm bath (about 10 minutes) followed by cool sponge and vigorous rub, given one or twice daily—put to bed afterward.
   b. Alternate hot and cold to the body, hot foot bath, cold compress to the head.
   c. Neutral wet sheet pack (p. 42).
   d. Cool saline enema. *CAUTION:* not tap water!
   e. Light diet, plenty of water, hot lemonade.
   f. Avoid noise, excitement, visitors.

3. Precaution—If the child is subject to convulsions, call the doctor while instituting above treatment vigorously. Consult doctor if fever does not lower, if fever persists more than twenty-four hours, or if other symptoms develop.

Bibliography

Books by Ellen White, available at Adventist Book Centers and at Adventist libraries:

Child Guidance
Counsels on Diet and Foods
Counsels on Stewardship
Counsels to Parents, Teachers and
        Students
Education
Healthful Living
Ministry of Healing
Selected Messages, Vol. II
Steps to Christ
Testimonies for the Church, Vols. I-III

Books — Available from medical libraries or publisher.

Life and Health. Bernell E. Baldwin. December, 1972. Pacific Press Publishing Association.

Stress of Life, The. Hans Seyle, Mc Graw-Hill, New York, 1976.

Taber's Cyclopedic Medical Dictionary, p. 377

Webster's Dictionary.

Index